DR. SEBI MEDICINAL HERBS

Healing Uses, Dosage, DIY Capsules and Where to Buy Wildcrafted Herbs

----

Remedies, Detox Cleanse, Immunity, Weight Loss, Lungs, Eyes, Nail, Skin and Hair Rejuvenation

By

Kerri M. Williams

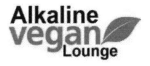

www.alkalineveganlounge.com

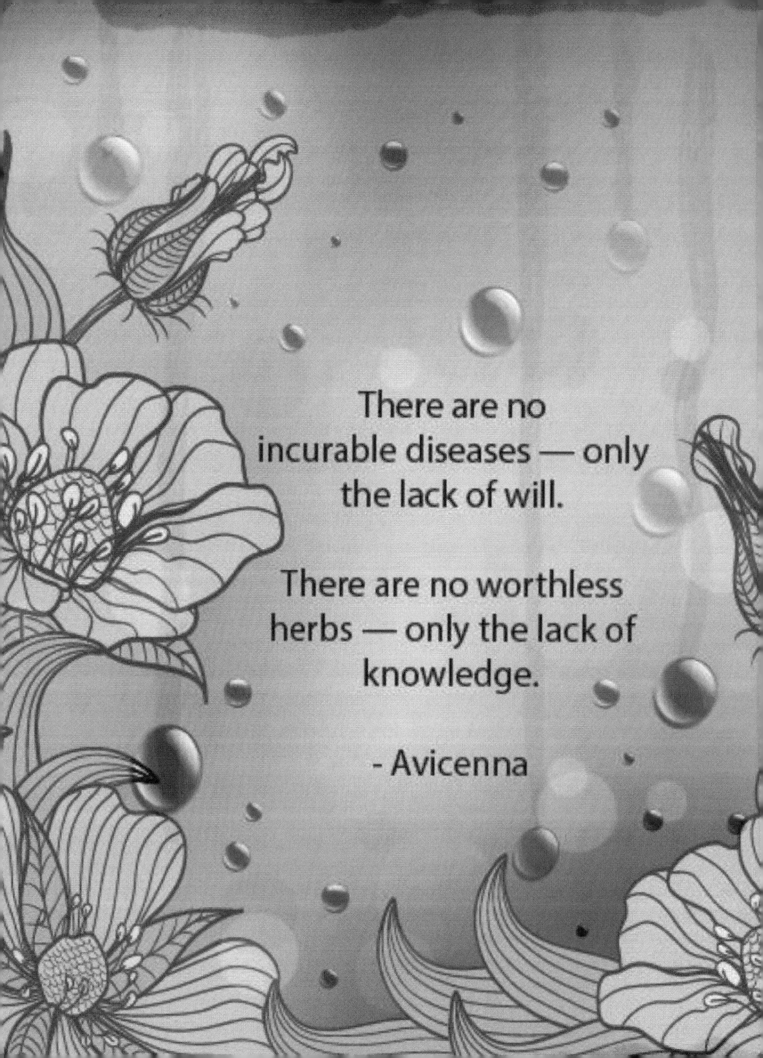

CONTENTS

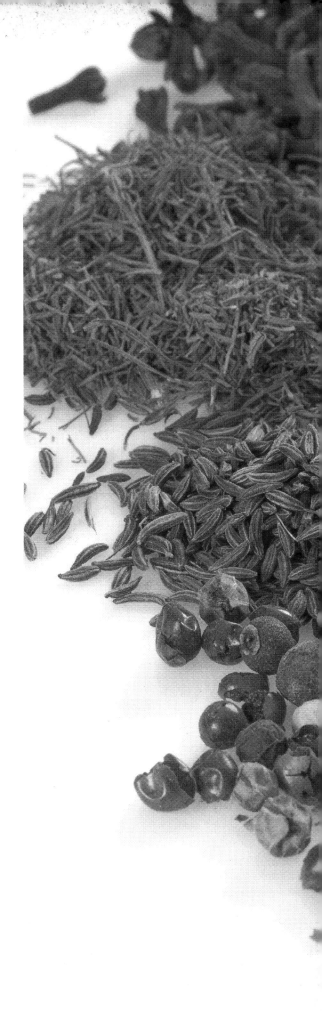

- **1 INTRODUCTION**
  - 3 Pharma vs Farmer

- **5 WHY ELECTRIC HERBS?**
  - 6 Proving that herbs work
  - 7 Herbal/Drug interactions

- **9 MEDICINAL HERBS**
  - 9 What are Herbs?
  - 13 The Plant Parts
  - 15 Sacred Herbs
  - 15 Herbal Medicine

- **19 SOURCING HERBS**
  - 20 Sourcing Herbs
  - 21 Storing Herbs
  - 21 Harvesting and Drying Herbs
  - 24 Wildcrafted Herbs
  - 25 Wildcrafted vs Organic Commercially grown
  - 28 Where to Buy Original and Organic Herbs

29 ENCAPSULATION AND DOSAGE

- 30   Tablets vs Capsules
- 31   Types of Capsules
- 32   How to Encapsulate Herbs
- 34   Preparing Herbs for encapsulation
- 35   How to Take Herbs as Capsules
- 35   How Much Cleansing Herbs to Take?
- 36   How to Prepare Herbs

40 SEBI APPROVED HERBS

- 40   Black Walnut Hull Powder
- 40   Bladderwrack
- 41   Blue Vervain
- 44   Burdock Root
- 45   Cascara Sagrada
- 47   Chamomile
- 48   Chaparral
- 49   Contribo
- 51   Damiana
- 53   Dandelion Root
- 55   Elderberry

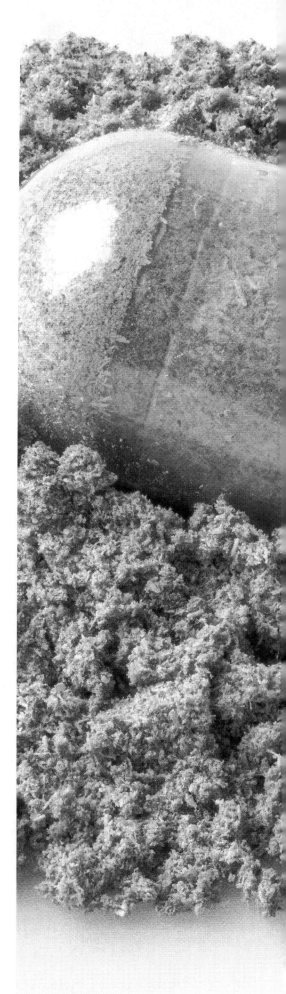

57	Irish Sea Moss
59	Kalawalla
60	Linden Flower
61	Lupulo
62	Nopal
65	Prodigiosa
67	Red Clover
69	Rhubard Root
70	Sarsaparilla Root
71	Soursop
72	Valerian Root
72	Yarrow
73	Yellow Dock

75 USING HERBS

76	Infusion vs Tea
79	Culinary Use of Herbs
82	Herbs for Topical Use
86	Smokable Herbs
87	Herbs commonly used for smoking blends
89	How to make your own smoking blend

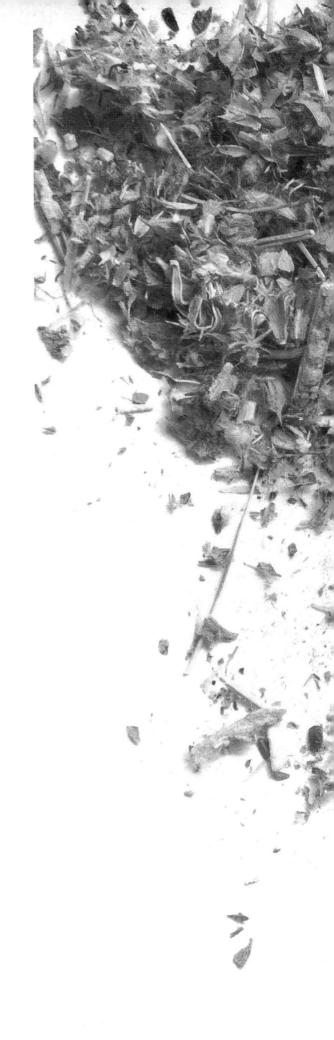

91 HERB COMBINATIONS

92 Herbs for Pancreas and kidney Support

95 Herbs for Liver Support

97 Herbs for Respiratory Support

99 Herbs for Colon Cleanse

100 OTHER BOOKS IN SAME SERIES

WWW.ALKALINEVEGANLOUNGE.COM

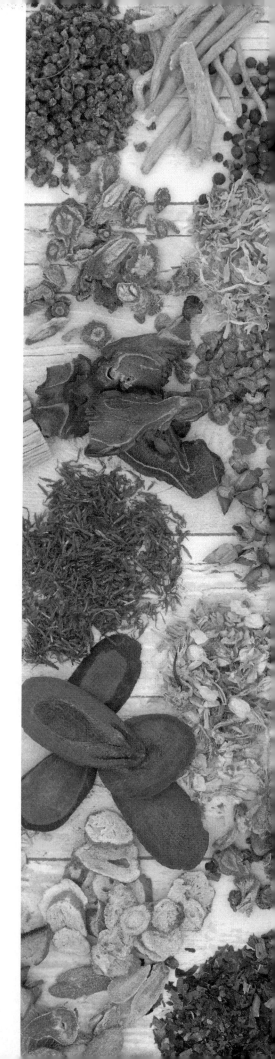

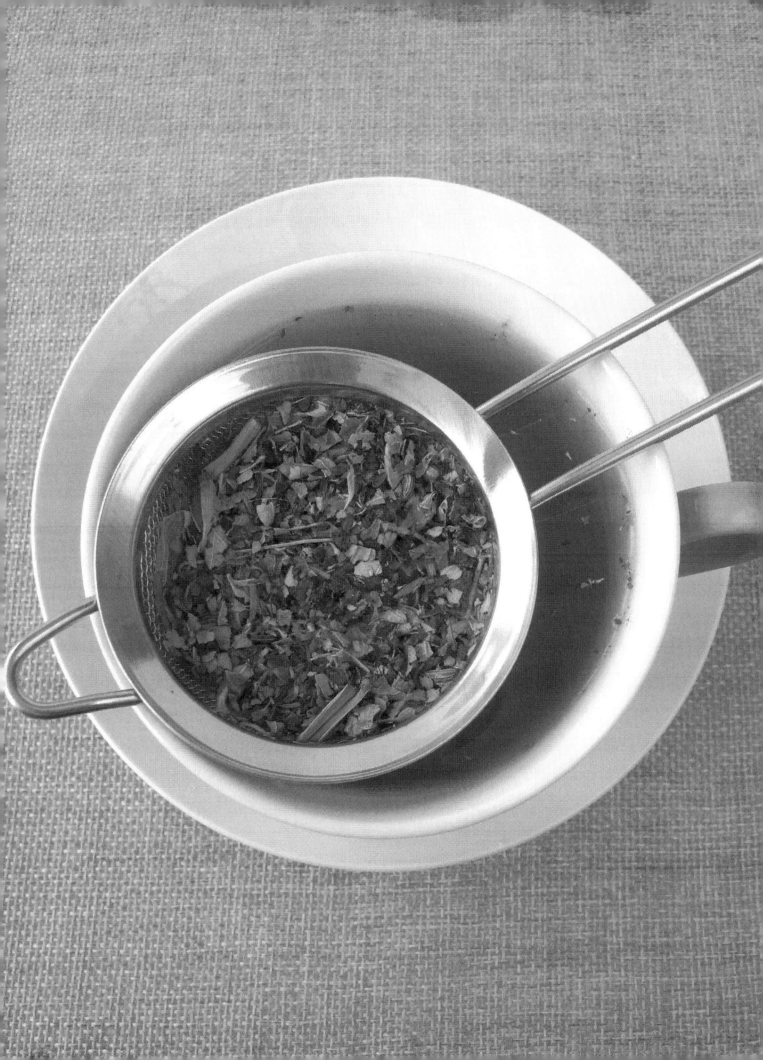

Copyright 2020 by Kerri Moon Williams

All rights reserved. Except as permitted under the U.S. Copyright Act of 1976, the scanning, uploading and distribution of this book via the internet or via any other means without the express permission of the author is illegal and punishable by law. Please purchase only authorized electronic and paperback editions, and do not participate in, or encourage electronic piracy of copyrighted material.

This publication is designed to provide competent and reliable information regarding the subject matter covered. However, it is sold with the understanding that the author is not engaged in rendering professional or nutritional advice. Laws and practices often vary from state to state and country to country and if medical or other expert assistance is required, the services of a professional should be sought.

Disclaimer:

The information provided in this book is for informational purposes only. Please consult with your health care provider for medical advice. The author specifically disclaims any liability that is incurred from the use or application of the contents of this book.

ABOUT THE BOOK

Hi and Welcome!

I so so love drinking herbal teas. Never a day that goes by, without having my warm drink of herbal tea. In fact, I'd give anything for having a warm herbal tea after workout! I cannot tell enough what herbs has done for my health and overall wellbeing. I was able to successfully reverse hypertension and maintain a normal blood pressure using herbal medicine. I have also improved my overall health, lost weight and live happy. I now have a better mood and disposition. Dr. Sebi alkaline herbs have so many benefits and one of the best ways I have noticed is to take them as teas. Herbal teas have replaced my morning coffee, it is my daily tonic. They have aided me in reversing diseases and maintaining optimum health.

In the course of my journey to healing, I researched and used Dr. Sebi herbs. For greater understanding, I have compiled them in the simplest and easiest way to understand. I really hope you get great value from it and helps you in your quest for healing and a healthier body. You can use these herbs in so many ways – either as an addition to smoothies, as tea (my favorite), taken in capsule form, or use as an ingredient for other benefits such as for tinctures, infusions, and beauty products. Consuming one herb at a time and watching out for how it makes you feel can make all the difference between what's great for you and what isn't. It's also great to learn more and read more books and also try out things for yourself, as with self-experience, you'll determine what's best for you.

If you are just getting started non the Dr. Sebi Diet lifestyle, and don't know how to begin, please check out my other books. Or if you have any disease such as diabetes or high blood pressure, you can learn how I SUCCESSFULLY LOWERED HIGH BLOOD PRESSURE in my book".

Furthermore, if you are completely new to the Diet, and would want to learn more on the Dr. Sebi's healing methodology and the African Bio-mineral Balance, you have a handy guide in several resources I have documented. You can also get a ton of resources on my website www.alkalineveganlounge.com.

Thank you once again for getting here. It is my sincere hope that you gain true healing and knowledge of that which you seek.

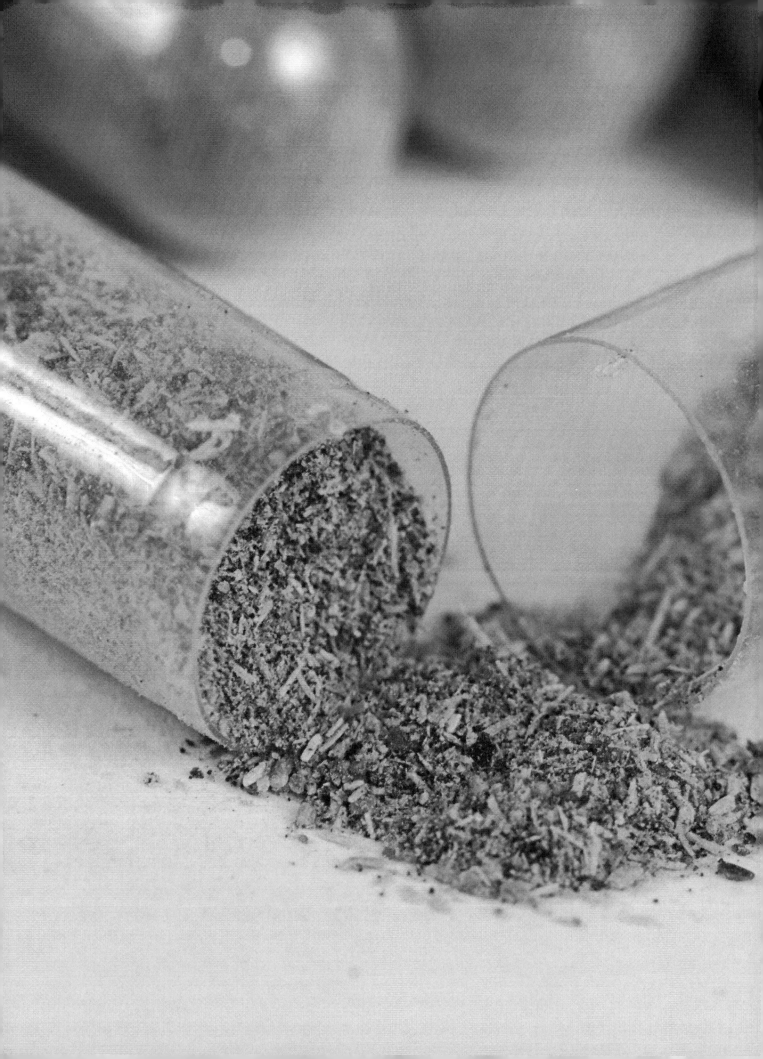

INTRODUCTION

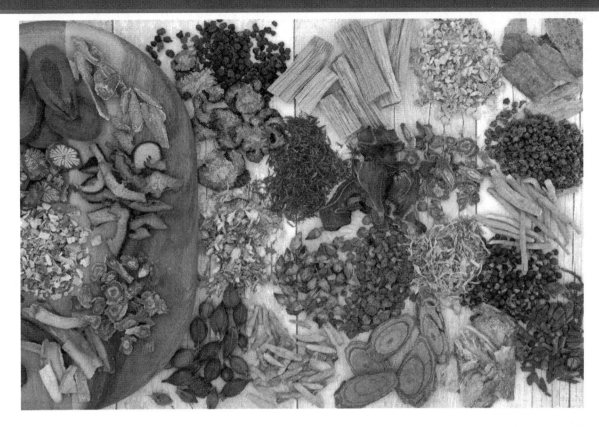

Over the millennia, many different healing traditions emerged around the world and all of them were based on herbalism. The major herbal systems were often drastically different from what most of us know as "Western herbalism" and it has taken us a very long time to "decipher" the meaning and understand the concept of some of the ancient holistic systems such as Ayurveda, Traditional Chinese Medicine, Shamanic healing, etc. Today, we know that one of the ways to prevent a disease or recover from one, is through a diet and the alkaline diet is probably one of the healthiest diets there is. However, there is not a single alkaline diet and what made Dr. Sebi Alkaline Diet stand out, is that his methodology was based on both *alkaline foods* and *medicinal herbs*.

Dr. Sebi studied herbs from Africa, North and South America, and Europe and focused his research and healing methodology on acid/alkaline balance within a human body. However, he did not base his therapies only on alkaline foods. He went a step further. He was adamant that all hybridized herbs (and foods) should be excluded from a healthy diet. Dr. Sebi insisted that alkaline herbs are essential for health and vitality and was very passionate about which herbs support one's health and which ones don't. His approach to herbalism was based on a belief that only that which is natural, can be truly healing. Most of the foods available today (ie fruits, vegetables, herbs, spices, grains, etc) were at some stage cross-bred to improve the yield. The list of all hybridized plants is too long to mention but the problem with this is that some of the herbs not approved by Dr. Sebi are unfortunately touted in the health community to have amazing health benefits, eg Aloe Vera, Echinacea, ginseng, turmeric, ginger, garlic, mint, etc. Dr. Sebi insisted they are hybrid and acidic and should be excluded from diet.

Dr. Sebi based his approach on the simple premise that wild plants were created in God's laboratory, while hybridized plants were created in medical laboratories through cross-pollination and genetic modification. As a result, they have an incomplete molecular structure. They are acid-based and should not be consumed for the simple reason that they are unnatural. According to Dr. Sebi, hybridized herbs and foods are acid-forming and negatively affect the brain (eg mint), destroy cells by weakening their membranes (eg garlic). If you are trying to heal using Dr. Sebi methodology, you should stay away from them.

So, although Dr. Sebi Alkaline Diet is very restrictive, he made up for the very limited choice of fruits, vegetables, herbs, and grains by including some highly nutritious herbal remedies and supplements. We are witnessing a steadily growing interest in holistic medicine. This is partly because, being better informed, people are now aware of the negative side effects that prescribed drugs come with. On top of that, the long-term use of antibiotics has led to the development of antibiotic-resistant bacteria. Besides, both painkillers and antidepressants are addictive and you will gradually have to increase the dosage if you want them to "work." For these, and many other reasons, more and more people are hoping to find a cure for their health problems in natural remedies. The technological innovations enabled us to have a glimpse into the amazing world of plants and to begin to understand how they interact with the environment and with the human body. They work both internally and externally and heal on all levels – physical, mental, and spiritual. They can destroy microbes, bacteria, and fungi. They reduce inflammation, dull the pain, help you relax, or boost your mental clarity. Some can induce vivid dreams or an alternate state of mind.

And, the most amazing thing of all is that many of these medicinal herbs with almost magical properties grow all around us and we often refer to them, and treat them, as "weeds".

PHARMA VS FARMER?

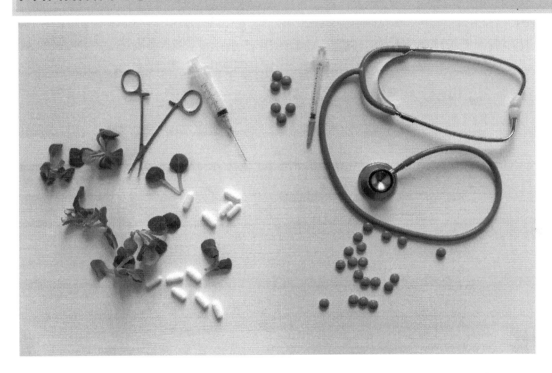

In the world we live in today, chronic diseases are on the rise, effectively making both conventional and alternative medicine a big business. And just when you realize that Americans spend more than $250 billion each year on drugs and supplements, then it is easier to understand how much of a problem the chronic disease pandemic has become. It's only human to want the best and safest, so we are naturally attracted to choose "quick fixes" – and worry about the side effects later. Be it food, drugs, herbs or supplement, we simply want the best – for health and healing. But the fact that what we see or hope to get isn't the reality is worrisome. Asides the benefits of synthetic drugs and pills, many Americans often go with supplements because they believe its healthier, costs less, and has little side effects. We have often been told herbal medicine is unregulated, and hence may be potentially more dangerous, but what about prescription drugs? Notwithstanding the side effects of drugs, we are made to believe that the cure is in the pill.

However, recent prescription drug recalls, have left much to be desired. *Zantac*, a popular H2 receptor blocker that treats extreme cases of acid reflux and heartburn, was recently pulled off the shelf. Zantac was linked to Stomach cancer and many other drugs with similar mechanism of action were also implicated. Other drugs such as Accutane and Vioxx were not spared – in fact, *Vioxx* in particular resulted in nearly 30,000 deaths and was used by more than 20 million people in a little over a 4-year span. These recalls and many others have further cast a doubt on not just conventional medicine, but the regulatory agencies including the U.S. Food and Drug Administration (FDA). But when you realize that the majority of Americans perceive the FDA's approval of drugs and food as a guarantee of safety and that all approval is based on "high degrees of certainty and clarity about a drugs benefits and risks", then you realize we may have a much bigger problem than we ever imagined.

So, when we look at all these, it begs the pertinent question – Can we really trust the conventional medical industry to getting true holistic health and healing? Can we continue to put our health on the line for silly errors or slippages? How long can we continue to swallow every pill and hope our health get better? I don't know. But what I do know is that soon, soon enough, a major paradigm shift will occur. We will realize all these and I hope it's not too late by then. I hope it is not too late to go back to mother nature and use her medicine that is bequeathed us.

CHAPTER 1
WHY ELECTRIC HERBS?

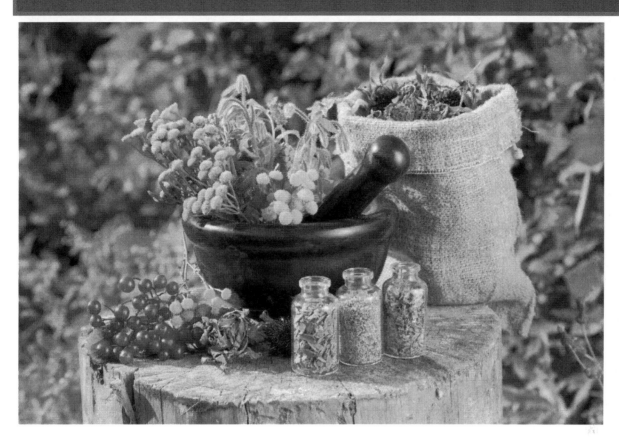

Electric Herbs are medicinal plants which helps the human body to heal, rebuild and nourish itself. They are alkaline and found in nature. They are not hybrid, irradiated, or genetically-modified.

Electric herbs improve the electrical activity in the nerves and helps with better cognitive function. It boosts your mental clarity and use of one's senses. Electricity is the reason the human body can move - crawl, walk, climb or run. Without electricity, there would be no movement and no life.

If the body is electric, then you should feed it electric (alkaline) nutrition. Electric herbs are herbs made in nature, non-hybridized and non-GMO. Electric herbs are wildcrafted, grown without the use of chemical fertilizers and pesticides.

PROVING THAT ALKALINE ELECTRIC HERBS WORK

There are countless people taking herbs that swear by their efficacy. Although many supplements and herbs are effective and safe, health science has been slow to confirm health claims. While pharmaceutical companies spent billions of dollars on drug research and discovery, herbs and other natural nutritional supplements often don't command big cash for research because they cannot be optimized to get a fiscal payoff the same way pharmaceuticals would. That notwithstanding, many adherents prefer and stick to natural herbs because of its natural healing properties and far less side effects.

Many herbs work pharmacologically as well as by action, providing a strong rationale for their use in healing especially where we have no alternatives in synthetic drugs. Note that many of the conventional synthetic drugs treat symptoms and hot heal. In other words, alternative medicine from nature's herbs will have true holistic healing compared to drugs. Picking between drugs and herbs is tough for so many people because the advice they will need to make these conclusions is mostly inaccessible. To date, there are only few clinical trials where the closest herbal medication was contrasted to a pharmaceutical drug and a placebo control.

With this, the I formation out there is limited and often confused. Aside healing uses and benefits, confusions often arise form:

Dosage - How much should I use?

Usage/Application – How should I use it?

Safety- How safe is this for me?

Sourcing – Where can I buy wildcrafted herbs

Contraindications – I am pregnant, would this be safe?

HERBAL/DRUG INTERACTIONS

Many herbs have been used to treat certain ailments for centuries. But simply because a product is organic or has been in existence for quite a while, that does not mean that you should assume that it is safer than pharmaceuticals. The same as interactions involving drugs, many herbs may cause adverse reactions when combined with medication or other nutritional supplements. A recent study published in the Journal of the American Medical Association demonstrated that one of prescription drug consumers, one in six adults chooses one herbal nutritional supplement together with a prescription medication, and many are unaware of the effect one could have on another.

This lack of information could have serious consequences. By way of instance, the popular memory booster sweeteners taken with aspirin can lead to bleeding, and St. John's wort, a popular remedy for depression, may negate the efficacy of oral contraceptives in addition to protease inhibitors used in the treatment of HIV. People who have existing health conditions, and pregnant women or people intending to conceive, have to be particularly conscious of drug/herb interactions, and talk with their doctors prior to making supplements part of the wellness plans, as they want prior to taking a prescription medication.

It is essential to be mindful of some interactions between herbs and pharmaceuticals. Also talk to your Physician before adding supplements to your health regimen, just as you would for a prescription medicine.

CHAPTER 2
MEDICINAL PLANTS AND HERBS

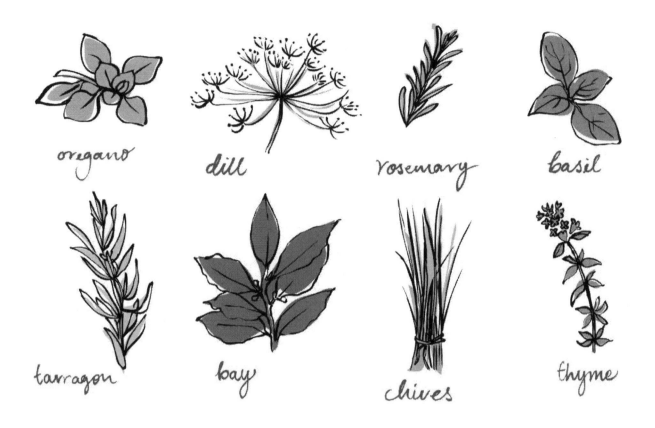

Herbs are not ordinary plants. They carry fragrance and aroma. They can be medicinal or sacred. They can flavor your food and environment. They can lift you up when you are down or calm you when you are anxious. And most importantly, they can heal.

WHAT ARE HERBS?

Herbs are usually only the green or leafy part of a plant (ie leaf, stem, and flower). On the other hand, medicinal plants (including those approved by Dr. Sebi) often use other parts of a plant, eg root, bark, berry, fruit, etc. Besides, there is a difference between herb and spice although many spices are often called herbs, eg cinnamon, etc. These two words are often used interchangeably and many plants that are actually spices, eg cumin, are often listed under medicinal herbs.

Common spices include:
1. Cinnamon
2. Paprika
3. Cayenne pepper
4. Peppercorn
5. Nutmeg
6. Cumin
7. Cardamom
8. Cloves
9. Fennel seed

However, regardless of how you call them and classify them, plants are essential for our survival. Not only do they provide food, housing, and building material, they also absorb carbon dioxide and release oxygen so we can breathe. Plants also help keep our waters clean. On top of all that, they nurture and heal.

The healing qualities of plants can be found in almost all their parts:
- Seeds
- Flower
- Gum/resin
- Leaves/sprouts/buds
- Bark
- Root
- Fruit
- Whole plant

- Sap
- Bean oil
- Rhizomes

When we speak of herbs, the first thing that comes to mind is the flavor they add to our food, however, they have many other uses, eg:

- **Domestic uses**

There are many ways you can use a herb around the house, eg basil keeps flies away, rosemary sprays deter mosquitos, a mixture of crushed cloves and lavender will protect your books and clothes from fish moths. Fresh herbs can freshen your house or you can make a potpourri with dried ones.

- **Cosmetic uses**

Herbs can resolve almost all your cosmetic problems, eg thin hair, discolored teeth, sagging skin, etc. They can infuse bath or massage oils or be used to make perfumes.

- **Medicinal uses**

Herbal remedies are usually taken as a tea, tincture, balm, infused oil, ointment, cream, essential oil, or Bach remedy. They are an effective alternative to many over-the-counter drugs.

- **Culinary uses**

You can add fresh or dried herbs to your meals or cocktails, or make an infused oil, vinegar, or butter. The possibilities are endless. So, if you disregard the plant/herb/spice division and treat the plants that can be used for healing, cooking, and cosmetics as herbs, you end up with a list of about 30 herbs, most of which have significant healing properties.

30 most common herbs:

1. Angelica
2. Anise
3. Basil
4. Bay leaf
5. Bergamot
6. Borage
7. Caraway
8. Chamomile
9. Chervil
10. Chives
11. Coriander
12. Dandelion
13. Dill
14. Elder
15. Lavender
16. Lovage
17. Marjoram
18. Nasturtium
19. Oregano
20. Parsley
21. Celery
22. Rosemary
23. Sage
24. Sorrel
25. Tarragon
26. Thyme
27. Yarrow

This is certainly not a complete list of medicinal herbs as there are hundreds of herbs that are difficult or impossible to grow commercially (eg those coming from the Amazon or from the semi-desert regions of Africa) or that are available only locally (eg most Ayurveda herbs, Traditional Chinese Medicine, South American herbs, etc). Not to mention the little-known herbs used by isolated communities in Australia, Siberia, etc. This may sound unbelievable, but new species of plants are still being discovered. They are usually found in remote places that had only recently been studied. Besides, new technologies make it possible to understand the biology of plants in a way that was not possible ten years ago.

THE PLANT PARTS

There are over 300,000 species of plants and regardless of how different their size, shape, and color may be, most of them have some things in common:

- **Root**

The root is the part of a plant that's located underground (or underwater). It is through the root that the plant draws water and minerals from the soil. Root also serves as an anchor that keeps the plant steady and in one place. There are different types of roots but the common plants usually have primary, secondary, and tertiary roots which represent the taproot system.

- **Leaves**

Leaves are organs of the stem. Their main function is photosynthesis, ie the conversion of carbon dioxide, water, and UV light into sugar (eg glucose). These simple sugars are processed into various macromolecules that are essential for the survival of the plant. The leaves transport these sugars to the roots and shoots and in that way support their growth. As sun and light are essential for photosynthesis, the leaves are shaped and located in such a way to ensure maximum exposure to sunlight.

Leaves are usually located above ground although some species have leaves underground (eg bulb scales) or underwater (eg aquatic plants).

- **Flowers**

The main function of flowers is to look and smell irresistible. Unless they can attract insects, birds, or animals, there'll be no one to pollinate them and ensure their survival. This is why plants have bright colors, strong scents, and sweet nectar. Combined, these attract pollinator who, by visiting many flowers, help move pollen from one plant to another. After pollination occurs, the flower develops seeds,

- **Stem**

The main function of a stem is to carry water and nutrients from the root to all other parts of the plant. With some plants, stems store the food, provide support, and enable vegetative propagation. Some plants have underground stems. Other plants develop stems with thorns that protect them from predators. Underground stems of some plants (eg strawberry or grass) spread and produce new plants when the old plants die.

- **Bark**

The bark is the outer covering of woody plants. Its main function is to preserve water and protect the plant from extreme temperatures as well as disease and predators. Some trees have such a thick bark that it can protect them from forest fires. Severe bark damage will kill the tree.

SACRED HERBS

Another important function herbs play in our life is that many of them are used in religions. For example,

- Hellenistic religion used myrrh and frankincense
- Anglo-Saxon pre-Christian religion used nine-herb charm
- In Hinduism, the sacred herbs are neem, holy basil (tulsi), and cannabis
- In Wicca (New Age), white sage is used for ritual cleansing both of one's aura as well as one's environment
- Some Native American tribes used white sage for spiritual cleansing
- Cannabis is the holy plant of Rastafarians
- Siberian shamans and Native Americans used herbs and hallucinogenic mushrooms to induce spiritual experiences

What's interesting is that all of these herbs have powerful medicinal properties and today, many are used for healing, eg cannabis, sage, tulsi, etc.

HERBAL MEDICINE

Herbal medicines are medicines made from plants that contain active ingredients. They may seem very gentle compared to conventional medicines but they still affect your body. This means that although they are natural, they should be used and prepared correctly or under guidance. Eight things to bear in mind before you attempt healing yourself (or others) with herbal medicines:

1. Some herbal medicines may interfere with the prescribed

medication (eg they may reduce or enhance the effects of conventional medicine). So, if you are on chronic medication, it's best not to take herbal medicines

2. If you have a serious health condition, eg liver or kidney disease and on chronic medication, you should not take any herbal medicine without discussing it with your doctor first. Besides, some herbal medicines may interfere with anesthesia or other medicines. For example, certain herbs may affect blood pressure or blood clotting which may increase the risk of bleeding during or after surgery

3. You may experience some adverse side effects, eg if you have an oversensitive digestive or nervous system, kidneys, skin, etc.

4. Don't start taking herbal medicines if you are about to have surgery. Or, if you are already taking herbal medicine, don't forget to mention this to your doctor

5. Pregnant or breastfeeding women should not take herbal medicine, nor should the elderly or children unless a qualified herbalist or your doctor were consulted first.

People relied on herbs for as long as they existed. Just like many animals look for certain herbs to eat if not feeling well, so people accidentally or through a trial-and-error method developed herbal medicine. There are written records that as early as 5000 years ago, Sumerians prescribed herbal remedies for many conditions.

What makes herbs healing, is the phytochemicals and phytonutrients they contain. These are compounds produced by all plants (some more than others). However, although herbs are natural, that doesn't mean they are harmless.

For example, St. John's wort and kava tinctures are well-known home remedies for depression and stress. However, if taken in large amounts or taken alongside prescribed medications, these herbs become toxic.

Besides, certain herbs contain psychoactive properties that have been used both for religious and recreational purposes, eg cannabis and coca plants. Archaeological and historical documents confirm that leaves of coca plants have been continuously used by the peoples of Peru for over 8000 years and that cannabis was regularly used in China and northern Africa as early as the first century CE.

CHAPTER 3
SOURCING AND/OR HARVESTING HERBS

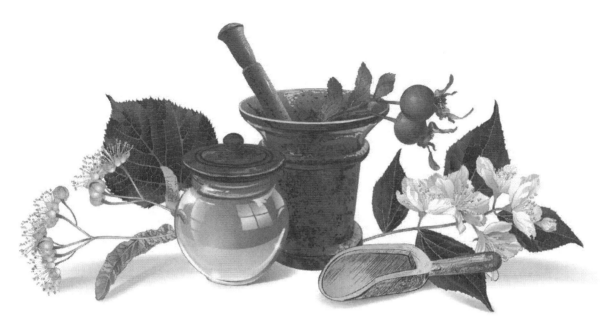

Before you can use herbs for healing, cosmetics, or food, you need to source them, dry them, and store them. As the awareness of the amazing therapeutic properties of herbs is growing, so is the demand for herbal remedies. To satisfy the needs of the growing population, herbs are now grown for profit. To increase the yield and protect their crops from pests, herb farmers use pesticides and herbicides that often contain harmful chemicals.

The problem with this is that these chemicals not only decrease a plant's nutritional value, they also negatively affect its medicinal properties. That means that, compared to wildcrafted herbs, farmed herbs give herbal remedies of inferior quality. In other words, instead of healing you, chemically-treated herbs add toxins to your already compromised body.

SOURCING HERBS

You can obtain herbs in three ways:

– **You can purchase them from a retail outlet**

This is usually not a good idea because retailers rarely have facilities for storing plant materials properly. In a retail outlet, herbs are usually kept in plastic containers, in open containers or sacs, and are not protected from light. Besides, as retailers deal with huge quantities, by the time they are sold, most of the herbs have lost their active ingredients.

It's safer to purchase herbs from small stores that order small quantities of herbs more frequently. How to know if a herb is fresh? If it has lost its natural color and has no fragrance, it probably no longer has any healing properties.

– **Order online**

Online orders are fine, provided you know who you're placing your order with. It's best to order from specialty companies as they usually store their herbs properly. Be careful when ordering from random sellers on Amazon. Please refer to the next section for a list of trusted online places to source approved medicinal herbs.

– **Grow your own**

Many herbs can easily be grown in a garden or in containers eg calendula, nettle, valerian, basil, etc. If your space is limited and you would like to grow your own herbs, it's best to choose herbs that grow vigorously and do not require a lot of space.

– **Buy from a local herb farmer**

If you happen to know a farmer who grows herbs, you will always have freshly-picked herbs.

STORING HERBS

The main reason herbs need to be stored carefully is that they contain volatile oils and plant pigments which are easily destroyed by light and damp. Besides, herbs easily absorb airborne pollutants, household air fresheners, cooking odors, smoke, etc which is why they should be stored in tightly closed dark-glass containers in clean and odor-free rooms.

However, before putting them away, you need to be sure they are dry otherwise they'll go moldy. If you have to store a herb that is still not completely dry, put it in a paper bag. Herbs usually retain their active ingredients for about a year (not more than 18 months) after which they should be discarded.

Fresh herbs should be washed, dried, wrapped in a paper towel, packed and thoroughly sealed in a plastic bag, and stored in the refrigerator for up to five days. Actually, herbs should not be washed because that destroys their volatile oils. However, as many people must have handled the herbs before they reached the market, it wouldn't be safe to use them without washing them first. Besides, they sometimes have soil, sand, insects, or fertilizers still attached to them. This is why it's so important to source herbs from reputable dealers.

HARVESTING AND DRYING HERBS

Improper storage can degrade herbs very quickly but their therapeutic properties can be destroyed even during the gathering. Herbs should be harvested on a dry, sunny day when their petals are fully open. Besides, most herbs should be harvested at the peak of maturity when the concentration of active ingredients is highest.

Harvested herbs should be dried as quickly as possible, ideally in a cool, dark, and drafty room free of dust, odors, pollutants, animal hairs, etc. That way you will preserve their flavor and active ingredients and prevent oxidation of other chemicals.

You can use an airing cupboard (leave the door open) or a damp-free garden shed. Never dry your herbs in a garage or a kitchen. In the garage, they would be contaminated with petrol fumes and in the kitchen, they would absorb the odors of frying, cooking, or baking.

Once they are dry, store them in clean, dry, dark glass or pottery containers with an airtight lid, out of direct sunlight. Alternatively, you can keep them in paper bags.

When to harvest and how to store various parts of plants:
- **Flowers**

Harvest after the morning dew has evaporated, on a sunny day but not during the hottest part of the day. Cut flower heads from the stems and dry whole on trays. If the stem is large of fleshy, eg mullein, remove the individual flowers and dry them separately. Some herbs should be gathered before they are fully open, eg lavender, borage, and chamomile.

- **Aerial parts and leaves**

Large leaves, eg burdock, can be harvested and dried individually while smaller leaves are best left on the stem. Leaves of deciduous herbs, eg basil, should be gathered just before flowering while evergreen herbs, eg rosemary, can be gathered or harvested throughout the year. When using all the aerial parts (flower, stem, leaves, and seedhead), harvest in the midst of flowering.

As a rule of thumb, leaves should be harvested before the plant flowers. Once they flower, leaves lose some of their flavor and become bitter, eg dandelion. Besides, when they are young and tender, leaves usually contain the highest amount of volatile oils which is what gives them fragrance.

- **Seeds**

Harvest entire seedheads with about 5 cm of the stalk when the seeds are almost ripe. You can hang them upside-down over a paper-lined tray or a tablecloth, or you can remove the seeds manually. Seeds should be harvested when fully ripe but before they become too dark, eg dill, fennel, coriander, caraway, etc.

- **Roots**

The best time to harvest roots is when the aerial parts of the plant have died down. Dandelion roots can be harvested in spring. Roots easily absorb moisture, so be careful where you keep them. If they become soft, throw them away. At the end of summer and beginning of fall, plants move their "essence" from leaves and flowers (which die down in winter anyway) to the roots. This is why roots should only be collected in the fall as that is when their therapeutic properties are highest, eg horseradish.

- **Sap and resin**

You can harvest these from the tree in autumn when the sap is falling. Make a deep incision in the bark or drill a hole and collect the sap in a cup tied to the tree. You can also squeeze sap from latex plants directly into a cup, eg wid lettuce, .

- **Fruit**

Harvest berries when ripe, before they become too soft to dry effectively. You can also spread on trays to dry.

- **Bark**

To minimize damage to the plant, the bark should only be harvested in the fall. Never remove all of the bark as that will kill the tree. Break the bark into smaller pieces and dry.

- **Bulbs**

Harvest only after the aerial parts have died down.

So, when to harvest herbs depends on which part of the herb you want to harvest, eg nettles in early spring, St. John's wort in summer, roots in the fall, some herbs throughout the year, etc. With some herbs, you take only leaves, eg basil, with others, you can take the whole herb. Generally speaking, it's also better to harvest herbs frequently as that will encourage the plant to produce new growth. Annual herbs can be harvested throughout the year until the frost kills them.

WILDCRAFTED HERBS

There is a huge difference between commercially grown and wildcrafted herbs. Whatever is commercial grown, ie fruits, vegetables, or herbs, was raised with the help of herbicides and pesticides. Besides, more and more plants are genetically modified which makes sourcing for healthy plants a real challenge.

2 main reasons wildcrafted herbs are superior to both commercially and organically grown ones:

- **Absence of toxins**

Wildcrafted herbs are those that grow wild. They are found in nature and, in an ideal world, they should be perfectly healthy. However, people often harvest and sell herbs collected next to busy roads. These herbs contain a lot of lead from petrol fumes as well as other harmful chemicals.

Many medicinal herbs look and are treated as weeds and can be found near roads, ditches, or rubbish dumps. So, although they grow wild and have not been treated with pesticides, many of the herbs collected in the wild have been "treated" with petrol fumes from nearby roads or pesticides and herbicides used by local farmers.

- **The potency of active ingredients**

Herbs growing in the wild have to cope on their own. There is no one to provide shade, water, protection from early frost, pests, and disease. However, the fact that they survived for millions of years suggests that they are either very strong or have developed resistance to environmental stressors and disease. Their nutrients and phytonutrients are their only defense against UV radiation, bacteria, fungi, and viruses.

So, when you use wildcrafted plants, you indirectly improve your own protection against these environmental stressors. In other words, the active ingredients of wild herbs are much more potent than those found in the farmed herbs. However, to ensure the survival of wild plants and herbs, it's essential that if you wildcraft, you follow the guidelines aimed at protecting both the plants and their habitats.

Guidelines for harvesting wild plants:
- Never harvest an endangered species
- Don't pick immature plants or unripe fruit
- Don't collect more than 15% of a particular plant in an area
- Don't harvest more plants than you need
- Don't damage surrounding plants or the environment
- Don't harvest from polluted environments

Unfortunately, not everyone has access to an unpolluted environment or to the wilderness, so the next best option is to grow your own herbs. Although space is often a problem, with a little bit of creativity, you can easily grow many herbs at or around your home or apartment. You can try:
- Container gardening
- Vertical gardening
- Windowsill gardening
- Rooftop gardening

WILDCRAFTED VS ORGANIC VS COMMERCIALLY GROWN HERBS

If you happen to have access to commercially grown, organic, as well as wildcrafted herbs, you may be at a loss which ones are best. This depends on what you're looking for.

- **Commercially grown**

Commercially grown herbs are cheap and available throughout the year. But, food grown for profit is farmed with very toxic chemicals. Until about a hundred years ago, farmers grew the food according to what the environment allowed and they foraged for herbs and berries.

However, with the post-war industrialization, mass production became an opportunity to make money quickly. The pharmaceutical industry came up with ways how to protect your crops from pests and increase yield. Greenhouses and cold storage made it possible to grow herbs regardless of the environment you live in and regardless of the time of the year. This was an opportunity for farmers and the pharmaceutical industry to make a lot of money – at the expense of our health.

Spraying pesticides and adding herbicides to the soil makes farming a lot easier and the yield more predictable, but over the years, this practice led to many serious diseases, eg asthma, allergies, nerve damage, some types of cancer, and many other conditions. And, unfortunately, washing herbs does not remove the toxins. What's worse, the pesticides are not only killing us, they are killing the bees and other beneficial insects necessary for pollination.

- **Organic**

Organic herbs are grown commercially but in controlled environments. They are raised on unpolluted land without the use of chemical fertilizers or herbicides. However, there are two problems with organically-grown herbs.

One is that being free of environmental stressors, eg drought, freezing temperatures, UV rays, etc, organically grown herbs are too "cushioned" from the environment which makes them weak. In other words, they develop their nutrients and phytonutrients without struggle since someone else (ie the farmer) is making sure they always have water, shade, medicine, etc. This reduces their nutritional and therapeutic value.

Another problem is that although you may be raising organic herbs without any chemicals, the water you use to water those plants is probably full of toxins, as is the air which they breathe. This varies from region to region, but it's becoming increasingly challenging to produce anything organic these days simply because our environment is so polluted. So, even if you live in a "clean" area, wind and rain will eventually pollute your crops too.

- **Wildcrafted**

With so many toxins and pollutants in our environment, wildcrafted plants should be harvested only from rural or remote regions. But, how many of us have access to such regions? Besides, even if you know of such places and know which herbs grow there, you need to know when particular herbs are ready to be harvested and be at the right place at the right time. This is possible but would require a lot of planning.

So, it's pretty self-explanatory what sort of herbs you should source if you want to reduce your toxic load.

WHERE TO BUY ORIGINAL AND ORGANIC HERBS

Below is the list of online places to buy organic herbs from:

Dr. Sebi Website (https://drsebiscellfood.com/products/)

Mountain Rose Herbs (https://mountainroseherbs.com/)

Starwest Botanicals (https://www.starwest-botanicals.com/)

TY Kitchen (http://tysconsciouskitchen.com/shop)

Alkaline Meal Ideas (https://allnaturellhealing.com/

The Sebian Shop (https://shop.thesebian.com/categories/alkaline-herbs

OTHERS

https://alkalineeclecticherbs.com/categories/alkaline-herbs

https://ahealthycrush.com/alkaline-herbs/

https://sebisdaughters.com/shop-2/

Recommended on Amazon

https://www.amazon.com/Premium-Irish-Moss-Superfood-Ounce/dp/B07BNSR49Q/ref=sr_1_37?dchild=1&keywords=best+sea+moss&qid=1604906372&sr=8-37

https://www.amazon.com/Black-Seed-Oil-Vegetarian-Cold-Pressed/dp/B0714PK8VV/ref=sr_1_33?dchild=1&keywords=Dr.+sebi+sea+moss&qid=1604906262&sr=8-33

https://www.amazon.com/Capsules-Express-Clear-Empty-Vegan/dp/B07X6KT8LC/ref=sr_1_6?dchild=1&keywords=vegetarian+capsules&qid=1604906957&sr=8-6

CHAPTER 4
ENCAPSULATION AND DOSAGE

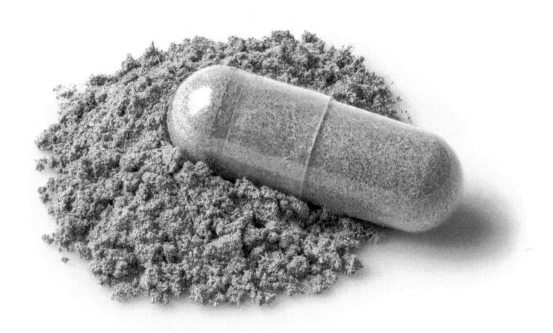

Oral medication can be taken in different ways (eg tea, tincture, oil, etc) but tablets and capsules are the most common ones. Although these two types of medicine delivery are very similar, there are significant differences in how they are made and how the drugs they contain are absorbed by the bloodstream. How much of a certain herbal remedy you should take depends on many things, eg on how you take it (eg tea or tincture), on the condition you are addressing (eg acute or chronic, mild or severe), your age (children and adults require different dosage), your overall health (are you a relatively healthy individual or is your immune system heavily compromised), etc. If you want to take herbal remedies in a powdered form, you usually take hen as tablets or capsules. Encapsulation is the process of turning medicine into a capsule.

TABLETS VS CAPSULES: WHAT'S THE DIFFERENCE?

There probably isn't a single person that has never taken a pill. Tablets are made by compressing one or more powdered ingredients into a hard pill. Besides medicine, tablets also contain additives that help keep all the ingredients together, and that improve the taste.

Tablets

Once swallowed, the tablet gets broken down in the digestive tract and the medication it contains is absorbed by the bloodstream. From the bloodstream, the drug travels to the liver from where it is sent to the target area(s). Tablets are inexpensive, long-lasting, can provide a higher dosage of medication, can be split, are chewable (in case you can't swallow), and come in quick-release, delayed-release, or extended-release formats. However, they are more likely to irritate the GI tract and are generally slower acting than the capsules.

Capsules

Medication found in capsules is enclosed in a shell. The absorption by the bloodstream and distribution throughout the body is similar to that of a tablet. The main advantage of capsules over tablets is that they break down more quickly which means you will experience relief from the symptoms sooner than you would if you had taken a tablet. Besides, they have a higher bioavailability (ie they are more effective than tablets). Unfortunately, their shelf-life is shorter, they are more expensive and usually come in small doses (ie you need several capsules to get the same effect you would get from a single tablet).

So, how to take herbal remedies and how much to take depends on many things, eg

- **Condition being treated**

Flu, depression, toothache, warts, sprain, insomnia, etc

- **The form of medication**

Oral or topical, dry or liquid, etc.

- **The type of medication used**

Applied to the skin, held under the tongue, inserted into the rectum, drops put into the ear or eyes, etc.

However, there are some general guidelines when it comes to taking herbal medicine, eg:

- **Tea**

Take 1 cup three to four times a day

- **Capsules**

Take 2-4 capsules two or three times a day.

- **Tincture**

1 teaspoon two to three times a day.

- **Tablets**

1 tablet two to three times a day.

TYPES OF CAPSULES

Herbal capsules are not difficult to make at home and if you have a chronic condition, you can save a lot of money by making rather than buying capsules. However, the main advantage of home-made capsules is that you know exactly what goes into them, you can be sure they contain no fillers or allergens, and you know they are freshly-made (as you won't be producing millions, but just a couple of dozen at a time). Besides, you can combine herbs in any way you want, ie your capsules will be unique.

Capsules can be soft gels or hard ones and if you want to fill your own, you should buy hard capsules. However, before you buy empty capsules, you need to have an idea of what you are going to fill them with, ie dry herbs or liquid medication. Besides, hard-shelled capsules may contain more than one drug which makes them ideal for dual-action or extended-release treatments. Soft gels are usually wider and the is medication held in a gelatine case.

Another classification of capsules is into gelatine based and vegetarian based ones:

- **Gelatin based**

Gelatine used to make capsules comes from cattle or pigs (the hoofs, bones, and connective tissue is boiled until it turns into a gel). Gel has certain health benefits, particularly for the skin and joints. This type of capsule is less expensive than vegetarian ones.

- **Vegetarian based**

These capsules are made of vegetable cellulose which comes from the bark of the pine and spruce trees. They are tasteless and odorless and ideal for vegetarians and vegans or for anyone else who cannot consume gelatin for any religious, cultural, or dietary reason.

Both types of capsules can be stored for many years without going off provided they are stored away from sunlight or heat. They should not be kept in a fridge for that will make them dry and brittle. Both types of capsules are ideal for storing powder or oil. They dissolve within 5 minutes after consumption.

HOW TO ENCAPSULATE HERBS

To start with, you need to purchase capsules. You can get either gelatin and vegetarian ones. You can ask for halal, kosher, gluten-free, BSE-and TSE-free ones.

Capsules are usually sold in bags of 500 or 1000 empty capsules. They come in different sizes which will determine which size of the encapsulation machine you should buy.

There are several sizes to choose from:
- "0" holds 500 mg of herbs. These capsules should be taken 2 per

day.
- "00" size holds 50% more herbs, about 750 mg. Being bigger, these capsules are more difficult to swallow.
- "1" size holds 400 mg and is usually used for making capsules for children or those who have difficulty swallowing.
- There are also size "2" (350 mg) and size "3" (200 mg).

Empty capsules can be bought from a local health food store or you can order them through Amazon.

However, to make your own capsules, you don't have to have a machine. You can encapsulate herbs by hand, but be warned - it takes time.

How to fill capsules manually:
- Pour the powdered herb into a small bowel.
- Open up the capsule.
- Use one half of the capsule to pour the herbs into another half.
- Close the capsule by pressing the two halves against each other.
- Repeat

However, if you plan to make hundreds of capsules or simply don't have time, you can get one of the encapsulation kits that can do 50-100 capsules at a time. Each of the kits is for a specific capsule size, so decide in advance what size capsules you want to make.
- Insert each end of the capsules into the respective slots
- Pour the powdered herbs into the machine. Move around until each capsule is filled (add more powder if necessary).
- Insert the top and close down until the capsules are "locked"

PREPARING HERBS FOR ENCAPSULATION

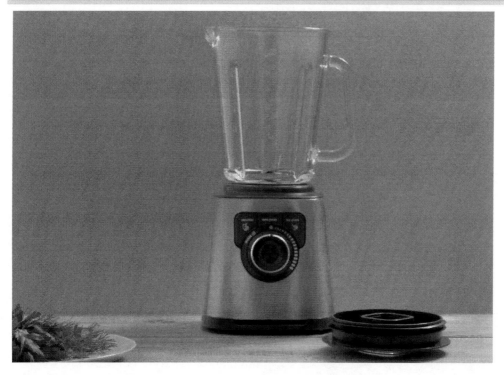

Preparing herbs for encapsulation starts long before they are packed into capsules.

6 steps to preparing herbs for encapsulation:
1. Harvest the herbs at the right time when their active ingredients are the most potent
2. Dry them properly so their volatile oils are preserved
3. Store them in a dry and cool place, away from light and heat
4. Buy the capsules
5. Grind the herbs into a fine powder (you can do this with a coffee grinder or with a mortar and pestle)
6. If you plan to use more than one herb, store grounded herbs separately and mix them just before encapsulation

CAN ALL HERBS BE TAKEN AS CAPSULES?

For a number of reasons, not all herbs are suitable for encapsulation. Those that are particularly easy to encapsulate include:

- Ashwagandha
- Black Walnut
- Cayenne
- Chlorella
- Damiana
- Horsetail
- Hydrangea
- Saw Palmetto
- Triphala
- Valerian root powder

HOW MUCH CLEANSING HERBS TO TAKE?

Just like every other alternative treatment, you should be mindful of the particular dosages to take when you take herbs. But one common problem with herbal remedies is the difficulty in determining the actual dosage to consume especially with raw herbs or roots. However, these have been made much easier with herbs that come in powder, granulated or capsule forms. With these, it's easier to take directly or make into herbal teas with specific ratios.

However, for full form roots, and chunks of stems, I usually recommend to research the actual dosage amount to take. For most herbs, it will need just a handful of herbs boiled in 10 ml of water.

For pre-made herb packages, simply follow the manufacturer's dosage instructions. If they do not come with instructions, the general rule to follow is 1 teaspoon part herb to I cup (8 ounces) of spring water. You can scale this ratio to make larger volume so you can store for use.

For pre-purchase cleansing packages –

Always follow the package recommended dosage or instructions on how you should prepare or take them. Most purchased packages come with instructions on how to take them.

For Leafy purchased herbs –

For leafy purchased herbs, this is determined as concentrations in ml. You can either prepare the fresh herbs directly by steeping/boiling a handful in 10ml of hot water or you can dry them and grind into powder form. Once ground, I like to measure 1 teaspoon per 8 oz (1 cup) spring water, which often is the general dosage rule for herbal mixtures.

Again, you can do additional research for the particular dosage of the specific leafy herb you want to prepare.

For bulk purchase herbs –

If you have purchased herbs in bulk and you're making your own teas, find out what the recommended dosage is for each herb. As a general rule, you should prepare each herbal tea in a ratio of 1 teaspoon to 8 ounces of spring water.

For capsules –

For herbs that come in capsule form, you should follow the recommended dosages for each herbal capsule.

HOW TO PREPARE HERBS

Preparing your cleansing herbs would depend a lot on the form you purchased them. Although, it's easier to prepare cleansing herbs that come in powder forms, as you can easily make herbal teas with them in the specified or recommended dosage. However, for other forms form herbs especially roots or leaves, it is better to use a ratio of 1 teaspoon to 1 cup (8 oz) of spring water for each herb.

However, for easier batch preparation and storage, I recommend preparing herbs in batches of mixtures. That would mean mixing them up according to function and benefit (Please refer to Chapter 7). Again, this will depend how state of health and what minerals are most important for you. You can combine similar herbs with similar functions into a batch. Like our healer, Dr.

Sebi would say, *"If you want calcium, you know where to go to (sea moss), if you want Iron, you go to Burdock, and if you want a mix of both Iron and Fluorine, you go to Lily of the Valley"*.

In all, try not to mix more than 2 or 3 herbs together. Remember, these herbs are electric, and its best to preserve their organic carbon, hydrogen and oxygen nature as much as we can. Again, if you mix more than that, you may not get their accurate concentrations per ml of water, so try to limit it to 3, possibly 2.

For clearer understanding, you can use the following mix:

- Mix Colon and gallbladder cleansing herbs together
- Mix liver and kidney cleansing herbs
- Mix respiratory and mucus cleansing herbs
- Mix lymphatic and heavy-metal cleansing herbs.

Since these herbs perform a whole-body cleanse (not just colon) including the skin, eyes, colon, liver, lymphatic system and gallbladder, you can decide to choose how to combine them. Also, note that when you make larger batches of these herbs for storage, try not to make batches that last more than 7 to 14 days

For pre-purchase cleansing packages –

Please follow the recommended dosage or instructions that are provided for that cleansing package

For Leafy purchased herbs –

For fresh Green leafy herbs

- Place in spring water and boil on low heat for 5 to 7 min
- For dried leafy herbs, boil longer – 10 to 15 min

For Dried ground (or powder) herbs –

For dried ground or powder leaves or roots, mix in recommended ratios for the herb. Powder herbs are the easiest to mix in dosage proportions so you can simply follow the package instructions

For Chunks of Dried Root herbs –

If you've purchased chunks of roots or stems, you can prepare them in the following way:

- Cut or break up chunks
- Place in spring water and boil for 15 minutes
- Let cool and serve
- Alternatively, dry and grind them into powder form using a power blender and then encapsulate
- You can also prepare them in larger batches and place in jars to store in the refrigerator.

For bulk purchase herbs –

If you have purchased herbs in bulk and you're making your own teas, find out what the recommended dosage is for each herb. As a general rule, you should prepare each herbal tea in a ratio of 1 teaspoon to 8 ounces of spring water.

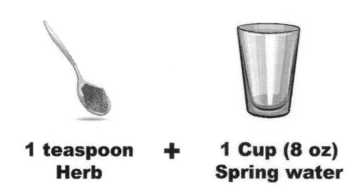

1 teaspoon Herb + 1 Cup (8 oz) Spring water

CHAPTER 5
DR. SEBI-APPROVED HERBS

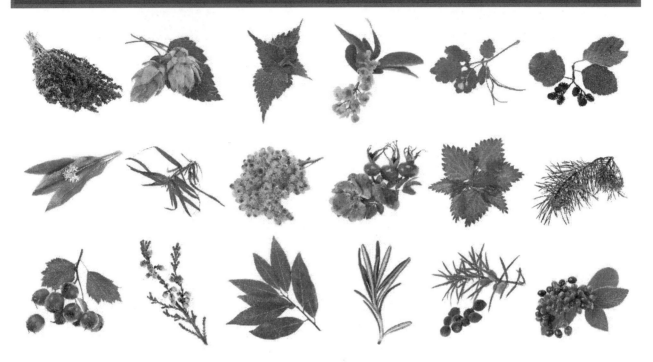

To Dr. Sebi, medicinal herbs were an essential part of his healing methodology but he was very particular about which herbs should be used alongside his alkaline diet. He was against all hybridized herbs as well as herbs that are not alkaline. In this chapter, we shall look at some of Dr. Sebi-approved herbs. Like most alternative medical practitioners, Dr. Sebi believed that prevention is better than cure. He taught us that an alkaline diet and herbal remedies could prevent or solve all our health problems. Dr. Sebi used the below-mentioned herbs to dry up mucus, free the body of toxins, and boost the immune system. This is a complete list of Dr. Sebi detox herbs and it contains herbs he recommended over and over again. In this chapter, we shall look at some of Dr. Sebi-approved herbs.

BLACK WALNUT HULL POWDER

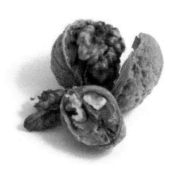
Black Walnut Hull (Fresh)

Black Walnut Hull (powder)

Description: Black walnut contains compounds that make it very effective in fighting bacteria and fungus. Besides, the tannins in black walnuts successfully dry up mucus and successfully kills parasites inside the body. This herb should not be taken on a regular basis, but only occasionally for cleansing. It can be taken as a capsule or a tablet.

BLADDERWRACK

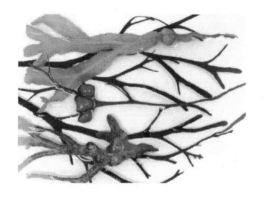
Bladderwrack (Fresh)

Bladderwrack (Dried)

Other Names: *Fucus vesiculosus*, Black tang, Bladder fucus, rockweed, Sea oak, Dyers fucus, cut weed, Rock wrack and Red focus.

Description: Bladderwrack is a found on the coasts the western Baltic Sea, the North Sea, and the Pacific and Atlantic Oceans. It is high in iodine – a key substance for thyroid health.

Uses: Used to take care of many thyroid ailments, e.g. underactive thyroid, outsized thyroid Gland, and potassium deficiency. It's also utilized for heartburn, arthritis, bronchitis, obesity, arteriosclerosis, digestive disorders, blood cleansing, emphysema, urinary tract disorders, constipation as well as nervousness. Other uses include boosting the immune system and increasing energy.

How to Use: Bladderwrack might be consumed whole, taken as tea or even blended with sea turtles from beverages and smoothies. To make tea, then combine 1 teaspoon per cup of warm spring water, and then allow to sit for 15 minutes prior to drinking. This may be taken one or two times every day.

Caution: Bladderwrack may potentially contain high levels of potassium, which might worsen some thyroid issues, so avoid protracted high or used doses.

BLUE VERVAIN (*Verbena officinalis*)

In pre-Christian England, vervain was considered a sacred herb. The ancient Romans also considered it sacred and used it to purify their homes and temples. It was regularly used in magic and ritual.

Blue vervain active ingredients include:
- Volatile oil
- Bitter glycosides
- Tannins

Dr. Sebi valued this herb very much and prescribed it for many conditions.

Medicinal properties of blue vervain:
- Relaxant tonic
- Promotes milk flow
- Stimulates labor
- Promotes sweating
- Nervine
- Sedative
- Antispasmodic
- Liver stimulant
- Laxative
- Uterine stimulant
- Urinary cleanser
- Fever remedy
- Bile stimulant.

Aerial parts should be gathered in summer while flowering. Vervain is usually taken internally but can be used topically as well.

Ways to use vervain:
- **Infusion**

Take for insomnia and nervous tension or to encourage sweating in the case of fever. Can also be used as a liver stimulant to improve appetite and digestion. If sipped during the labor, it will encourage contractions and if taken during lactation, will stimulate milk flow

- **Tincture**

Use for depression, as a stimulant for liver, nervous exhaustion or for poor digestion. It can be used in combination with other urinary herbs for stones and conditions related to excess uric acid

- **Poultice**

Apply to muscle sprains, insect bites, and bruises

– Ointment

Use on skin problems such as eczema or wounds. Can also be used for neuralgia

– Mouthwash

You can use the infusion for spongy gums, or mouth ulcers

Caution:
- Avoid the herb in pregnancy. This is because it stimulates the uterus. However, it may be taken during labor as it stimulates contractions

BURDOCK ROOT *(The Efficient Blood Cleanser)*

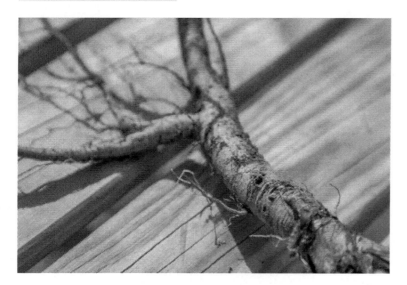

HISTORY: Burdock was used as far back as the middle ages to heal several disorders. They have been used by early herbalists to relieve pain and purify the bloodstream from China, India and Europe.

DESCRIPTION: Burdock Root comprises all 102 minerals which form the human body in trace quantities.

KEY BENEFITS: Assists with indigestion, joint pain, detoxifying the liver, and balancing hormones. Helps improve skin quality, decrease inflammation, and reduce blood glucose levels. USES: Heal insomnia, cancer, Gastrointestinal ailments, joint pain, arthritis, kidney infections, complications of syphilis, & skin ailments such as psoriasis. May assist with gout, thyroid health, bladder ailments + kidney & gallbladder stones.

TASTE: Getting a nutty sweetness and taste

HOW TO USE: Blend it with Dandelion Root to get a great "java" or into Perrier + Date Syrup to create a "beer. I love to blend it with other herbs to provide me a nutrient increase. Since Sarsaparilla is greatest in iron and behaves as a magnet for the rest of the minerals, I blend them frequently (typically with a 3rd herb which rounds out the taste (such as Linden Flower). CAUTION: If You've Got a Bleeding disease, burdock may increase bleeding.

CASCARA SAGRADA *(The World's Natural Laxative)*

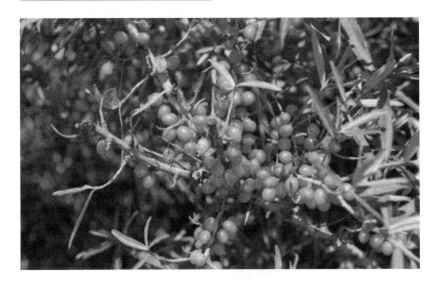

Other names: Rhamnus Purshiana, Bitter bark, Sacred bark, Cascara buckthorn, Bearberry, chittem rod and chitticum stick

Variants: None

History/Origin: The bark of Cascara Sagrada was used as far back as the 1600s from the natives of the Pacific shore and Euro-Americans as a natural laxative. It was also used as one of many anthraquinone-containing herbal medications. Commercially it's known as "Cascara sagrada" (meaning 'sacred bark' at Spanish), though, traditionally it's called "Chittem bark" or "Chitticum bark". Spanish soldiers moving round the Pacific Northwest struck many natives utilizing the bark for a laxative and gave it the title "sacred bark" with regard to its own efficacy.

Description: Considered a high All-natural laxative by herbalists. It's supposed to be the best herb for colon cleansing accessible. Cascara sagrada is proven to serve as a natural antibiotic in the intestines when taken internally. It's been used to eliminate gastrointestinal ailments such as worms.

How it functions: Cascara sagrada will cause a bowel movement over eight to 12 hours taking a dose. It induces muscular contraction in the gut which help move stool throughout the gut. Additionally stimulates the liver/pancreas secretion.

Cascara sagrada increases the secretion of bile in the gallbladder. As a result of this property, it's been used to divide and prevent gallstones.

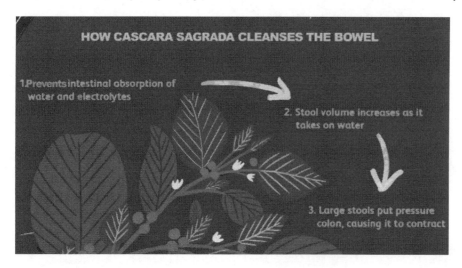

Key benefits: Laxative for constipation, therapy for hepatitis, liver disorders, and also cancer. A colon cleaner thought to enhance the muscular tone of the colon walls.

Other applications: It Is believed to ease the strain and pain associated with hemorrhoids and anal fissures too (however this claim is just supported by traditional use).

Taste: It does not taste great.

How to utilize: Cascara sagrada will generally cause a bowel movement within 12 hours, so it is Ideal to take it at night in order that at the morning it is simpler to use the bathroom

Caution/Side Outcomes: Can cause laxative dependence since the intestines start to adapt to this anthraquinones and be able to operate by themselves. Please refrain from accepting it for more than two weeks without needing a rest (at least two days). Don't advise

Drinking this and then heading out for a very long amount of time in which you must use a toilet in somebody else's home.

CHAMOMILE

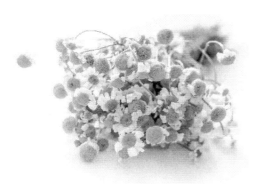

Chamomile (Flower, fresh)

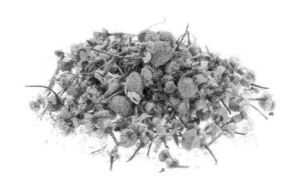

Chamomile (Flower, dried)

The plant is indigenous to Europe and has been used for centuries for medicinal purposes. Ancient Egyptians worshipped it for its incredible healing powers. It has a soothing effect on your skin and calming effect on your mind which is why it is used for skin conditions or as a tea to help you get a good night's sleep.

Chamomile boosts your immune system by helping your sleep well because when you're well-rested, your immune system works better. It is usually taken as a tea to reduce muscle tension and anxiety, to improve digestion, relieve stomach cramps. It has a powerful sedative effect and if you have trouble sleeping make a strong brew before going to bed. You can wash your face with chamomile tea or pour strong chamomile tea into your bath to relieve sunburn. Use only loose-leaf chamomile, never teabags.

CHAPARRAL *(The Anti-Inflammotory Herb)*

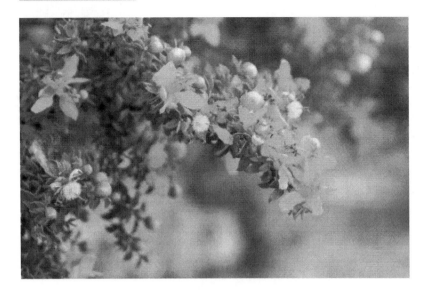

Other Names: Larrea divaricate, Creosote bush, Hediondilla, Greasewood, Jarilla, zygophyllum tridentatum. Variants: Larrea tridentate, larrea divaricata, larrea Mexicana

History: Chaparral was reported to be as old as 4 million years of age. Chaparral originates in the creosote regions, which will be a desert tree native to southern area of the USA and northern portion of Mexico.

Description: Chaparral is a yellow flowering plant using quite bright blossoms and dark green leaves. All areas of the plant have been used for medicinal purposes but despite its own usage, it's quite controversial and was reported to be prohibited in certain states including Canada.

Key Benefits: This cleanses the lymphatic system and stomach. Also will help to clean heavy metals in the blood and reduced blood glucose levels.

Uses: Employed to deal with insomnia, cancer, skin disorders, arthritis, and STDs

Taste: Chaparral includes a sour flavor with a rather strong taste.
Caution: No significant side effects; although could lead to skin irritation when applied to the skin

CONTRIBO *(Aristolachia grandiflora)*

This herb is known by many other names, eg Bejuco de Santiago, Dutchman's Pipe, Calico Vine, Vine of St. James, Liana couresse, Six Sixty-six, Pipe vegetale, Tref, Twef, Birthwort, and Trefle caraibe.

This unusual plant has a huge flower that smells like rotting meat. We mentioned earlier that plants have to have attractive flowers and a strong scent in order to attract bees, birds, and insects who will pollinate them. As contribo flower is pollinated by a fly, it shouldn't be surprising it developed a smell of rotting meat as that is the smell flies are most drawn to. Throughout Central America, contribo is a popular natural remedy for colds and flu, stomach ache, and indigestion. It can also be soaked in rum and used as a bitter.

Contribo is a jungle-vine that needs to be sun-dried before it becomes a medicinal herb. The dried vine is then soaked in water or liquor. The liquid is drunk as and when necessary, and new liquid is added to replace the consumed liquid. It should be kept in a cool, dry place.

Contribo is usually found in wet areas and is a well-known medicinal herb not only in Central America but also in western herbal medicine, Ayurveda, and Traditional Chinese Medicine (TCM). Apparently , it's been used for its therapeutic properties since 300 BCE.

Conditions that can be treated with contribo:

- Kidney problems
- Bladder stones
- Stones
- Gout
- Snakebite

- Uterine complaints
- Insomnia
- Skin conditions (eg bruises, wounds, skin infections)
- Alleviate fever
- Enhance appetite
- Strengthens the immune system

Contribo can be used as a tea or its powder can be mixed with honey and olive oil. It can also be used topically as a lotion to treat wounds and skin infections.

Although this herb has been known and used for a very long time, there have been very few scientific studies of this plant.

Unfortunately, contribo doesn't come without side effects so it's best to use it under the guidance of a qualified herbalist.

Caution:
- Due to aristolochic acid, continuous use of contribo can have very negative effects on one's health.
- It contains high amounts of calcium oxalate, so overuse could lead to kidney stones

DAMIANA (TURNERA DIFFUSA)

Damiana is a shrub native to Mexico, Texas, Central and South America, and the West Indies. It has been used as a herbal remedy for a very long time. By the time the Spanish colonized South America, indigenous peoples had been using it for centuries.

There is very limited scientific research on this herb

Damiana is also known by many other names, eg Damiana Herb, Damiana Aphrodisiaca, Old Woman's Broom, Damiana Leaf, Feuille de Damiana, , Damiane, Feuille de Damiane, Houx Mexicain, Mexican Damiana, Oreganillo, Mizibcoc, Rosemary, Turnera aphrodisiaca, Thé Bourrique, Turnera diffusa, Turnerae Diffusae Folium, Herba de la Pastora, Turnera diffusa var. aphrodisiaca, Turnera microphyllia and Turnerae diffusae herba.

Active ingredients of damiana relate to the endocrine and nervous systems. It is used both to relax the body and boost energy levels.

Damiana medicine is made from the leaf and the stem. It can be used as a juice, tea, or supplement (capsule or tincture). Damiana herb can also be smoked or inhaled as it mimics the effects of marijuana.

Medicinal uses of damiana include:

- Treatment for obesity
- Improved mental and physical performance
- Immune support
- Natural remedy for asthma
- Natural remedy for diabetes
- Relieves headache
- Reduces depression and anxiety
- Stomach complaints
- Relieved constipation
- Fights infections
- Relieves symptoms of menopause and premenstrual syndrome

complaints
- Acts as a bladder tonic
- Helps you get "high"
- Acts as an aphrodisiac (improves libido)

Caution:
- Pregnant and nursing women should not consume damiana, nor should anyone with liver conditions
- Damina leaves are safe to smoke or inhale but in high doses can cause hallucinations

DANDELION ROOT (*The Great Coffee Replacement*)

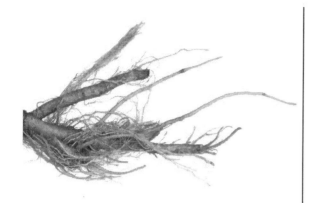
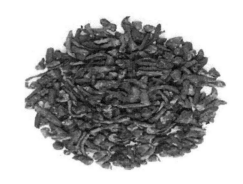

Dandelion (Root, Fresh) | Dandelion (Root, Dried)

Dandelion Root

OTHER NAMES: Lentodon taraxacum, Blow-ball, Bitterwort Cankerwort, Common dandelion, Clockflower, Irish daisy, piss-in-bed, Lion's tooth, Pissinlit, Puffball, Priest's crown, swine's snout, Yellow gowan, Telltime.

VARIANTS: None

HISTORY: Dandelion was a well-known recovery plant for centuries. They have been popular in ancient Egypt, Rome and Greece and also have been utilized in their conventional medicine. Dandelions likely came in America by travellers that used it for medicinal advantages.

DESCRIPTION: Even though a Fantastic coffee substitute, Dandelion is an awesome herb for liver-cleansing. Cleansing the liver provides you some energy back. Thus, drinking it in the morning is a superb java substitute and allows the entire body to stay in detox mode rather than getting all of the acid that coffee drinking could create within the body.

KEY BENEFITS: This amazing Herb may improve your immune system, destroy free radicals, combat diabetes, and help with sinus ailments, and even combat cancer. Additionally, it enhances energy levels; alleviates stomach upset, intestinal gas, gallstones, joint pain, muscle aches, & eczema; and utilized to treat viral diseases.

USES: It's been used to deal with Viral diseases and improve immunity. Reduces inflammation and cholesterol; reduces blood pressure, also helps regulate glucose levels.

HOW IT WORKS: Its curative Impact in the liver also helps cleanse the bloodstream that assists in clearing up skin conditions such as psoriasis, eczema and psoriasis.

TASTE: Dandelion Root Tea Tastes much like java, so there is no excuse to not give up coffee for your wholesome lifestyle. Insert Hemp Milk and Date Syrup and you have got the healthiest latte in history

HOW TO USE: You are able to consume the Flowers, leaves, stalks, and also the origin. The whole plant may be utilized in salads, soups, and vegetable dishes.

CAUTION: In some individuals, Dandelion might lead to stomach distress, diarrhea and heartburn.

ELDERBERRY *(The Great Immunity Booster)*

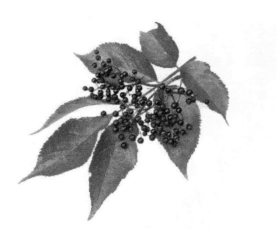
Elderberry (Herb, Fresh)

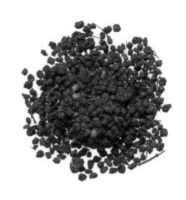
Elderberry (Herb, Dried)

OTHER NAMES: Elder, Common Elder, Black Elder, Black-Berried Alder, Black Elderberry, Bountry, Boor Tree, Baccae, Baises de Sureau, Arbre de Judas

VARIANTS: None

Elderberry have been used for since the seventeenth century for a wide range of ailments. It was majorly used by the people of Northern Africa and ancient Asia to wade of evil spirits and cure several health problems.

DESCRIPTION: Used medicinally by herbalists to boost the immune system during cold and flu season. Almost every part of the elder plant has medicinal or culinary value. Dr. Sebi focused on berries as studies show they have antioxidant, antidiabetic, anti-inflammatory, and immune-modulating, as well as antidepressant properties. Elderberries are high in nutrients. They contain flavonoids, vitamins (A, B1, B2, B6, B9, C and E), minerals (K, Ca, and Mg), as well as phytochemicals (eg carotenoids, phytosterols and polyphenols). Elderberries are successfully used for respiratory, cardiovascular, and mental health. As it has strong anti-viral properties, it is most often used to fight the symptoms of flu.

KEY BENEFITS: anti-inflammatory, antiviral, anti-influenza & anticancer properties. Used to boost the immune system. Aids the healing process, stimulates digestion and eliminates chronic pain. It is also said to possess chemo-preventive properties.

USES: Packed with antioxidants they help to cleanse the body, improve vision, speed up the metabolism, increase respiratory health, lower inflammation, and protect against chronic disease.

HOW IT WORKS: Elderberry helps loosen mucus from the upper respiratory tract and lungs, making it easier to cough up mucus, which in turn prevents respiratory infection from resulting to bronchitis or pneumonia

It also helps with increased perspiration via sweating and urine flow.

TASTE: Although elderberries don't taste sweet, they have a somewhat mild earthy taste with a tart flavor

They can be used to make a great combo with other herbs so as to make them more palatable.

HOW TO USE: It's best not to eat raw elderberries as they contain some cyanide. They can be cooked and used to make juice, jelly, syrups, wine, smoothies or in salads (cooked). The most popular way is to make it into a syrup or to use as infusion in teas.

If you can't take the herb, you can take in capsule form, usually about 3 capsules per day.

CAUTION: Avoid taking elderberries as regular berries. They can cause often result in diarrhea, nausea or vomiting if taken raw.

IRISH SEA MOSS *(The Daily Mineral Intake Companion)*

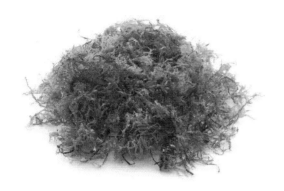

Irish Sea moss (Fresh)

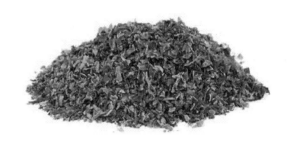

Irish Sea moss (flakes)

OTHER NAMES: Chondrus Crispus, Irish moss, Irish carraigín, carrageen moss, the tiny stone HISTORY: The title "Irish Moss" was originated through the potato famine in Ireland back in the nineteenth century. During the famine, many were hungry and desired food that was in short supply, then they resorted to eating the red alga that climbed on the stones.

DESCRIPTION: A Excellent species of algae That grows along the rugged areas of the Atlantic coast of North America and Europe. A fantastic daily vitamin supply. Includes 92 of 102 minerals which compose the entire body. Sea moss is an alga and is still a very fantastic source of dietary fiber, vitamin and several minerals (calcium, copper, iron, magnesium, phosphorous, potassium, phosphorus, sulfur, and manganese).

BENEFITS: aids in fostering the metabolism, encouraging the immune system, relieving joint pain, soothing the digestive tract, + supporting cardiovascular health.

HOW TO USE: To gain most from this herb, it is ideal to take it in conjunction with bladderwrack. Create a warm drink from it with hemp dates and milk. And try to drink twice or once daily preferably in the afternoon and day. I also use it to cleanse my Face many times every week. I just blend a dime sized amount of this powder with spring water, then make it into a paste, and spread it on my face. I leave it around for 5 minutes or longer, then wash.

Sea moss powder could quickly be utilized as an inclusion in smoothies, or add capsules or made in to gel. The powder form is simpler to use if you're just beginning, otherwise you might need to contend with the sea moss herb at which you'll first have to soak and

mix to make gel.

CAUTION: No known side effects

KALAWALLA *(The Natural Anti-Oxidant)*

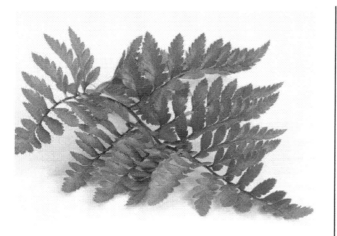
Kalawalla (Herb, Fresh)

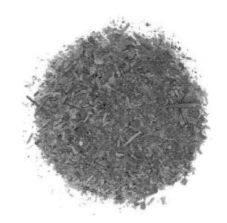
Kalawalla (Herb, Dried,

Other Names: Calaguala, *Polypodium decumanum,* Callawalla

Variants: None

History: From the jungles of Honduras, they grow exclusively over Palm trees in symbiotic relationship.

Key Benefit: antioxidant, immune system,

Uses: The indigenous people use it as a blood purifier. It contains three types of amino acids that are powerful antioxidants and protect your DNA from free radicals. Kalawalla is particularly effective for those suffering from skin conditions and has also been to treat neurological disorders like Alzheimer's.

Taste: more like a bland taste. Kalawalla does not have a bitter or after taste.

How to Use: For best results, take Kalawalla every day as a tea.

Caution: Very little or no side effects. Although some have reported a little indigestion and some skin rashes.

LINDEN FLOWER *(Natural Expectorant)*

Great for expelling mucus from the lungs. Really soothing. It's my go to if I have a dry throat or a persistent cough. It has a mild flowery taste. Wonderful addition to herbal blends for balancing out strong flavors.

KEY BENEFITS: Can aid in lowering blood pressure and inflammation. Gives relief to gastrointestinal discomfort and helps with efficient digestion.

USES: Used for colds, stuffy nose, mucus relief, sore throat, fever, breathing problems (bronchitis), and headaches (including sinus and migraine

HOW IT WORKS: It makes it easier to bring up phlegm by coughing (as an expectorant).

TASTE: A light, flowery taste. Good to mix with more bitter herbs to help balance out their taste.

HOW TO USE: Wonderful addition to herbal blends for balancing out strong flavors.

LUPULO

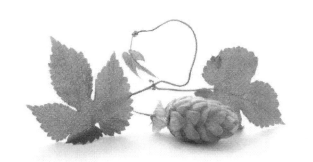
Lupulo (Herb, Fresh)

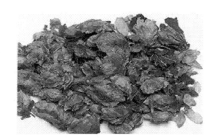
Lupulo (Herb, Dried)

Lupulo is a well-known natural remedy used to relieves pain. help to calm the nerves, improve sleep, help with hot flashes. By calming you down, it indirectly lowers your cholesterol as well as blood pressure. One usually takes these herbs for 7 to 30 days after a cleanse, detox or fast.

The longer you fast, cleanse or detox, the better. However, there is a limit to how long your body can go on without solid foods before it gets sick, so don't overdo it. Therefore, regardless of how you decided to heal your body, eg with a cleanse, detox or fast, as soon as you're done with it, start taking revitalizing herbs and follow the Dr. Sebi alkaline diet. Irish moss and iron can be consumed both during the cleanse and during the revitalization.

If you follow an alkaline diet, you should cleanse once a year for 7 days. Otherwise, for the best results, you should perform a cleanse every three months.

NOPAL *(Opuntia ficus cactaceae)*

Most people are probably unfamiliar with the word *nopal*, although most have heard of prickly pear cactus. Nopal and prickly pear are, in fact, the same plant. Nopal cactus originates in the deserts of the southwestern United States and Mexico. It is a common ingredient in Mexican cuisine but can only be eaten fresh when young (that's when the fruit is juicy and tender). Nopal fruit is also used to make marmalade, soups, stews, and salads.

Therapeutic properties of nopal revolve around its antiviral and antioxidant properties. There are over 100 species of nopal in Mexico and it has been used in traditional medicine for hundreds of years.

Some of the common medicinal uses of nopal:

- **Prevents viral infections**

Nopal cactus has antiviral properties and early studies suggest that it can be effectively used against herpes simplex, respiratory syncytial virus, and HIV.

- **Protects nerve cells**

When your nerve cells are damaged you end up with sensory loss or pain. Nopal cactus can protect against this damage

- **Protects cells from free radicals**

Being high in antioxidants, nopal protects your cells from damage caused by free radicals.

- **Regulates blood sugar**

Consistent use of opal cactus can regulate blood sugar levels. It is best if nopal is taken together with other diabetic medications.

- **Helps treat enlarged prostate**

An enlarged prostate makes you want to urinate more frequently. Nopal helps not only with an enlarged prostate, it is also used in prostate cancer treatments.

- **Helps reduce cholesterol**

Nopal cactus can help you lower the "bad" cholesterol with much fewer side effects than traditional cholesterol medications.

- **Eliminates hangovers**

Nopal cactus helps relieve the symptoms of hangovers but the problem is it should be taken BEFORE you start drinking.

You can benefit from the healing benefits of nopal cactus either by eating it raw or taking it as supplements (capsule, powder, or tincture).

Nopal juice benefits:

- Lowers cholesterol
- Antioxidant and anti-inflammatory properties
- Relieves pain
- Boosts immune system
- Protects the liver
- To treat bladder and urinary issues
- As an aphrodisiac

Conditions that can be treated with nopal:

- Glaucoma
- Wounds
- Fatigue
- Liver conditions

- Ulcers
- Diabetes

Caution

- Commercially produced nopal juice is often mixed with other fruit juices which means it usually contains much more sugar than the pure nopal juice would. So, anyone with diabetes should avoid taking commercially-produced nopal juice and should rather choose fresh fruit or freshly squeezed home-made nopal juice.

However, when buying nopal juice from street vendors, remember that most of them use tap water to rinse the fruit. Such juice is not pasteurized and treated for bacteria although cattle manure is used as a fertilizer. A recent study found that over 90% of street-sold nopal juice tested positive for *Escherichia coli* and 1% tested positive for Salmonella. If you love this juice, it's best to buy it from a reputable source.

- Nopal cactus has fewer side effects when eaten as food than when taken as a supplement. To be on the safe side, get your nopal from a reputable source. Potential side effects of nopal supplements include headache, nausea, and diarrhea

- Pregnant women should never take nopal supplements

- Nopal supplements can affect your blood sugar levels, so if you have diabetes you should be particularly careful. It's best to discuss this with your doctor first.

PRODIGIOSA

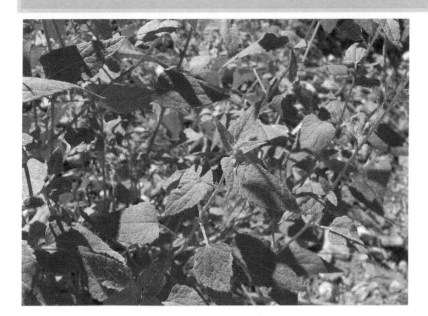

Other Names: Brickellia Grandiflora, Brickellia canvanillesi, Amula, Calea zacatechichi, Hamula, fantasy plant, Bitter bud, Cheech. Variants: Brickellia Grandiflora, Brickellia canvanillesi

History: Prodigiosa is a species of snout moth that originated from Peru.

Description: This really is a dark green bushy herb with leaves around the top side and a greyish purple color on the bottom. It develops as large as 5 feet. The flowers on this plant include a pure white color to a yellowish shade and may be seen growing in clusters. This perennial plant could be found flowering almost throughout the year.

Prodigiosa is frequently talked about as being correlated with all the dark arts because it had been used in voodoo for part of their rituals. But this herb is not difficult to cultivate and develops just too in a plant pot also. Its medicinal advantages shouldn't be overlooked and by developing this herb into your garden, you're never too much from a new cup of herbal tea.

Key Benefits: Prodigiosa arouses pancreas secretion, reduces blood glucose, and enhances fat digestion in the gall bladder. Helps with gut digestion, supports healthy kidney function, helps maintain Wholesome Glucose Levels, supports a healthy immune system

Uses: Immune system, Gallbladder and Pancreas, immune system health, reduces blood glucose, and is valuable for individuals with diabetes.

Taste: it's quite bitter in flavor.

You may think of this as a bad thing but when it comes to digestion, bitter is better.

How to Utilize: Take as tea or in capsule form. Once consumed as tea, then the herb produces lactic acid, which assists stomach digestion. Make tea by brewing leaves (fresh or dried) in warm spring water. Since pf the sour flavor of these leaves, you may add date syrup into it. This tea may be taken twice each day.

Caution: No known unwanted effects.

RED CLOVER (*Trifolium pratense*)

Traditionally, red clover was used as a fodder crop for cattle. It is only recently that we became aware of its health benefits.

Red clover active ingredients include:

- Phenolic glycosides
- Flavonoids
- Salicylates
- Coumarins
- Cyanogenic glycosides
- Mineral acids

Only the flowers have therapeutic properties and it's best to harvest them during flowering.

Effect it has on the body:
- Alterative,
- Antispasmodic
- Diuretic
- Anti-inflammatory
- Oestrogenic properties

Traditionally, red clover was used for skin complaints and to treat coughs and bronchitis but in the 1930s it was recommended to treating certain types of cancer, eg breast, ovarian, and lymphatic. Unfortunately, after the boom of the pharmaceutical industry in the 1960s, red clover is no longer considered an effective cancer treatment. Still, many holistic doctors prescribe it as an anti-cancer therapy.

7 ways to use red clover flowers:

1. Fresh flowers
Crushed fresh flowers may be applied to insect bites and stings

2. Tincture
Take internally for skin problems like psoriasis and eczema.

3. Compress
Use for arthritic pains and gout

4. Eyewash
Use about 6-12 drops tincture in about half an ounce (20 ml) spring water for a well-strained infusion for conjunctivitis or a full eyebath

5. Douche
Use the infusion for vaginal itching

6. Syrup
The syrup is an effective treatment for stubborn, dry coughs

RHUBARD ROOT *(The Natural Laxative)*

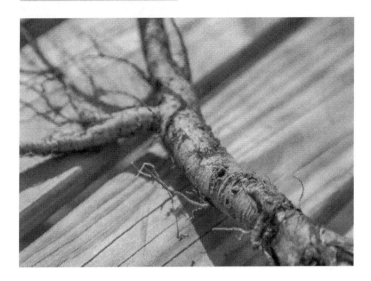

Other Names: Chinese Rhubarb, Garden Rhubarb, Da Huang, Himalayan Rhubarb, Medicinal Rhubarb, Indian Rhubarb

Variants: *Rhizoma Rhei, Rewandchini, Rhei, Rhei Radix*

History: The name "Rhubarb" was derived from rhabarbarum. Rhabarbarum's herbal uses started as far back as 5000 years ago, when Chinese used its roots as a laxative.

Description: Rhubarb has a distinctive yellowish root. Highly effective in improving the tone and health of the digestive tract, the root and rhizome (underground stem) are used as medicine.

Benefits: It also helps in cleansing the bowel of heavy metals and harmful bacteria. Helps relieve constipation, bloating and cramps

Uses: Used for digestive issues such as diarrhea and constipation; stomach pain, heartburn, ulcer or stomach bleeding, etc.

How It Works: Works mainly as a laxative

Taste: Has a sweet-sour taste with a tangy flavor.

How to Use: Use as tea

Caution: Can cause uterine contractions; should not be used if pregnant

SARSAPARILLA ROOT

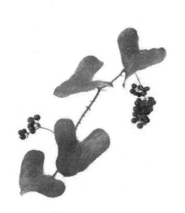

Sarsaparilla (Herb, Fresh)

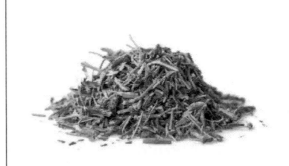

Sarsaparilla (Root, Dried)

DESCRIPTION: This is one of the very best natural resources of iron, a mineral necessary in the practice of recovery. It has diuretic and restorative properties.

Used for its Anti-inflammatory, antiulcer, antioxidant, anti-inflammatory, diaphoretic & diuretic properties. It comprises plenty of plant compounds believed to have a favorable influence on the body.
BENEFITS: Anti-inflammatory, Antiulcer, antioxidant, anti-inflammatory, diaphoretic & diuretic properties. Maximum concentration of iron of any plant.

USES: Assist with inflammation, congestive Heart failure, higher blood pressure, PMS, urinary problems, hypertension, migraines, nervous system disorders, and suffering from arthritis.

HOW IT WORKS: Compounds Called saponins might decrease joint pain and skin itching, and kill germs. May also aid in reducing inflammation and protecting the liver from harm. Maximum concentration of iron of any herb (based on Dr. Sebi).

SOURSOP (The Powerful Antioxidant)

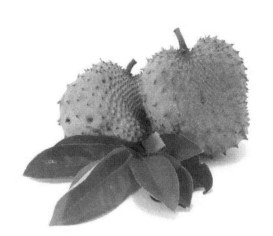
Soursop (Herb, fresh)

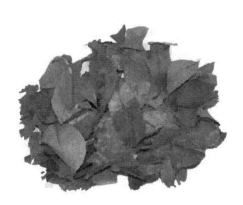
Soursop (Leaf, dried)

Other Names: Custard apple, Annona muricate, Guanabana, Brazilian paw, Cherimoya

Variants: None

History: Soursop Is a plant which grows in rain forests of Africa, South America, and Southeast Asia.

Description: It Comprises over 200 phytochemicals and contains anti-inflammatory and antioxidant properties. All areas of the plant possess medicinal properties.

Benefits: It can assist you to enhance the state of skin, nails and hair. High in carbohydrates.

Uses: It May Help Kill Cancer Cells, assist Fight Bacteria, decrease Inflammation, modulate Blood Glucose Levels

Taste: The Fruit includes a buttery sweet flavor while the leaves possess a spoonful of tartness

How to Use: You May take it as extract or tea but it's ideal to eat the leaves and fruit raw.

Caution: None

VALERIAN ROOT

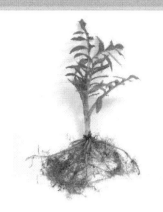
Valerian root (Herb, Fresh)

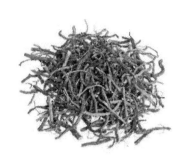
Valerian root (Herb, Dried)

An ancient remedy for anxiety, stress, nervous asthma, hysterical states, hypochondria, headaches, and stomach upsets. You can use it for hypertension caused by stress.

YARROW

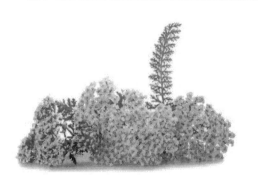
Yarrow (Herb, Fresh)

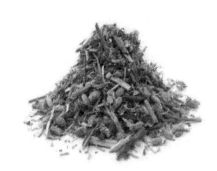
Yarrow (Herb, Dried)

Traditionally, it has been used to promotes sweating and stop wound bleeding. It can also reduce heavy menstrual bleeding and pain. Can ease gastro-intestinal problems, cerebral and coronary thrombosis, lower high blood pressure, improves circulation, and tone varicose veins.

YELLOW DOCK *(Rumex crispus)*

The dock is very similar to sorrel and has a multitude of medicinal uses. Native to Europe and Asia, it is now found throughout the world where it is often considered a weed. Both the leaves and the root have therapeutic properties. Leaves are also used in cooking.

Medicinal use of the yellow dock is based on a tincture, syrup, or an ointment. Ointments made to relieve itching and swollen glands, are prepared by boiling the root in vinegar and the pulp is then mixed with coconut oil or a similar agent. It is available in capsules and as tea.

Yellow dock active ingredients:
- Tannins
- Resins
- Salts
- Volatile oils
- Starches
- Thiamine

The yellow dock comes with many health benefits but was traditionally used to treat various skin conditions (eg ...) and as a mild laxative. It has astringent and purgative properties and has been used to treat many different conditions.

Conditions that can be treated with yellow dock:
- Poor digestion
- Liver detox
- Skin conditions (eg scabies)
- Inflamed nasal passages
- Rheumatism

- Scurvy and scrofula
- Constipation
- Promotes bile production
- In some parts of Africa, warm dock leaves are used to dress swollen breasts during lactation, and also pound and pulp the leaves for use as a pile treatment.
- Laryngitis and gingivitis (the dried root of dock mixed with warm water is used as a gargle to treat laryngitis, and as a mouthwash.it is also effective against gingivitis)
- Intestinal infections (eg ringworm)
- Fungal infections
- Jaundice

Caution:
- Yellow dock contains oxalic acid which can irritate the bowels and may cause mild diarrhea.

- You should not use yellow dock if taking drugs to decrease blood calcium, eg diuretics, Dilantin, Miacalcin, or Mithracin. Or if you have kidney disease, liver disease, or an electrolyte abnormality

- Overdosing on the yellow dock may cause metabolic acidosis – a very threatening blood disorder as well as calcium deficiency in the blood.

- The yellow dock should never be consumed uncooked as it may cause severe reactions. Even just handling raw yellow dock may cause a skin reaction in some people

CHAPTER 6
USING HERBS

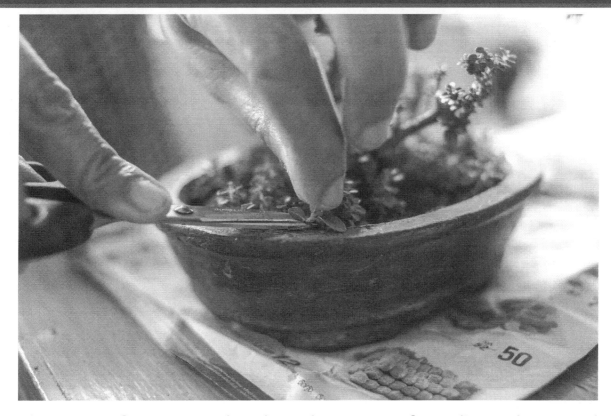

Herbs, in one form or another, have been part of our diet, culture, and medicine since time began. Herbs provide nutrition and medication. They affect our mood and emotions. They are part of many religious ceremonies and spiritual quests. They make our life and our environments more beautiful, refine, and liveable. But, it is the grassroots medicine that has kept us alive over millennia. Unfortunately, the art of self-care and preventative medicine has been lost as we embraced "development". But, whether we embraced it willingly and out of ignorance or were made to forget "the old ways" for the sake of modernity, is another question.

The fact is, more and more people are looking to nature in the hope of finding a cure for an ailment or to protect themselves against degenerative, incurable "diseases of civilization" (cancer, stroke, heart disease, autoimmune disorders, obesity, diabetes, etc). There are many ways to benefit from the nutritional and medicinal properties of herbs but the easiest ones are through tea, food, topical application, steam inhalation, and smoke.

INFUSION VS TEA

A herbal infusion and tea are, more or less, the same thing. Still, there is a difference in the way they are made and what they are used for.

2 main differences between tea and infusion:

- **The amount of herb used**

To make tea, you usually need 1 teaspoon of herbs to a cup of hot water. Water is poured over the herbs. Traditional tea is either black (Indian) or green (Chinese) while herbal teas are made from fruits, leaves, and flowers. To make an infusion, you use much more herbs (2-3 tablespoons per cup).

- **The steep time**

To make a cup of tea, you usually steep the herbs for 5-10 minutes (this depends on the herbs and on the strength you want to achieve). After steeping, you strain the herbs or remove the tea bags. Tea is usually taken warm.

To make an infusion, you can use either hot or cold water. Herbs are usually steeped for several hours, or in the case of the cold water infusions, overnight. Because it is steeped for longer, an infusion is often higher in nutrients than tea.

In other words, both infusion and tea are a process of extracting chemical compounds or flavor from a plant. But, neither infusion nor tea ever use boiling water. Water should be hot, just off the boil, otherwise, most volatile oils would be destroyed.

However, tea and infusion are terms that are often used interchangeably. The point is, certain plant nutrients only become available if the herb has been soaked in hot water for a long time. We now know that it takes at least four hours to get a significant amount of nutrients from the herb into the water. Roots and barks need to be seeped for at least 8 hours.

This may come as a surprise to many, but if you steep 2 teaspoons of nettle tea in hot water for ten minutes, you get about 5-10 mg of calcium. Also, if you steep 2 teaspoons of nettle tea in a liter of hot water for at least 4 hours, you get over 200 mg of calcium per cup (plus all the other nutrients the nettle leaves contain).

So, a long herbal infusion gives a beverage high in minerals, vitamins, essential fatty acids, and proteins. Such a drink also contains anti-cancer phytochemicals and antioxidants, as well as many nutrients essential for healthy bones, a balanced immune system, strong nerves, stable blood sugar, good digestion, etc. In fact, it is much more effective to take herbal nutrients through an infusion than through nutritional supplements. Liquids (eg infusion) is absorbed by the bloodstream without having to go to the stomach where some of the nutrients are destroyed by gastric acid.

Many professional herbalists will confirm that if used consistently, long infusions are a very efficient natural remedy for many conditions, eg osteoporosis, anxiety, adrenal burnout, eczema, diabetes, sinus problems, allergies, hormonal problems, infertility, joint pain, high blood pressure, etc. This is because long infusions provide large amounts of nutrients that cannot be obtained from teas or tinctures.

Long herbal infusions are believed to be one of the best (and easiest) ways to improve your overall health, eg your energy levels will increase, you will become more resilient to stress, you will sleep better because your body will have enough nutrients necessary for supporting a healthy nervous system, you will gradually even stop craving junk foods, etc. In other words, by choosing your plants carefully, with long infusions, you can easily add all the essential nutrients to your diet.

However, not all herbs are suitable for long infusion, eg St. John's Wort. Herbs that have very powerful sedative or stimulating properties, should never be prepared this way although they are perfectly safe to take as tea.

How to make a long infusion:
- Take 1 oz (28 grams) of chosen dried herbs (that's about 4 tablespoons)
- Place in a glass or ceramic jar with a lid
- Cover with one-liter hot water
- Stir and close tightly with the lid
- Let it sit for 4-8 hours (or overnight)
- Strain and refrigerate unless you plan to use it during the day. It will keep in the fridge for 48 hours. You can gently reheat it, add honey, milk, sugar, or salt and tamari (to nettles),

The best herbs to use for long infusion include:
- Red clover
- Nettles
- Violet
- Linden
- Chickweed
- Burdock root
- Dandelion root

These two last herbs are an essential part of the Dr. Sebi-approved alkaline diet. When used as a tincture, Burdock Root provides support for the menopausal symptoms eg hot flashes, night sweats, heart palpitations, increases vaginal lubrication, etc. It also helps you detox, stabilize blood sugar, and improve digestion.

A Burdock tonic can help you lose weight by improving your metabolism, reducing cravings, and strengthening a sluggish thyroid.

A Dandelion tonic can also help you lose weight by improving your metabolism, while Dandelion root remedies support the liver and make detox easier.

On top of all these health benefits, both Burdock and Dandelion leaves and root can be taken as long infusion, a process that intensifies their healing properties. No wonder Dr. Sebi was so passionate about these herbs.

CULINARY USE OF HERBS

When it comes to cooking, herbs are usually classified as woody (eg rosemary and thyme) or soft herbs (basil and sage). Woody herbs are tougher and come with a more powerful aroma and are usually not eaten raw. They are usually used to flavor a dish and are removed before the dish is served. Woody herbs taste better dried than fresh.

Soft herbs are very delicate and can be eaten raw in salads (basil) or drinks or used simply for decoration. They have a subtle flavor and are usually added only once the dish has already been cooked or are added during the last few minutes. You should never cook soft herbs (eg parsley, chives, sage, etc) as all their volatile oils will be lost in the process. It's best to sprinkle them just before serving. Some of the culinary herbs are very aromatic or colorful and scattering just a few leaves over a dish can have an amazing aromatic and esthetic effect. Soft herbs are best used fresh and you can easily grow your own, even if you don't have a garden.

The common culinary herbs include:

- Angelica
- Anise
- Basil
- Bay Bergamot
- Borage
- Caraway
- Celery
- Chamomile
- Chervil
- Chives
- Coriander
- Dandelion
- Dill
- Fennel
- Lovage
- Marjoram
- Mustard
- Nasturtium
- Oregano
- Parsley
- Rosemary
- Sage
- Sorrel
- Tarragon
- Thyme
- Watercress

Some of these also have therapeutic properties (eg oregano, thyme, dandelion, sage, fennel) but only if they are harvested, stored, and used properly. So, herbs can be used for cooking, garnishing, stuffing, or seasoning. They are also added to preserved foods, both sweet and savory.

Culinary herbs can be used to make:
- Soups
- Stocks and gravies
- Sauces and stuffings
- Salads
- Salad dressings
- For garnishing
- To add flavor to pasta or rice
- In puddings
- For baking bread
- In jams, jellies, and syrups
- To infuse oil or vinegar
- To add flavor to pickles
- As tea

The herbs mentioned so far are mainly those used in Western cuisine. The herbs and spices used in other parts of the world are often very different. Asian cuisine is particularly well-known for the variety of herbs and spices, many of which have well-known therapeutic properties, eg cloves, etc.

Some of the best-known herbs used in African and Asian cooking include:
- Cardamom
- Cloves
- Black pepper
- Cumin

- Coriander
- Nutmeg
- Curry leaf
- Mustard seeds
- Fenugreek
- Saffron
- Allspice
- Tamarind
- Star anise
- Chilli
- Cassia
- Sesame seed and oil
- Fennel seed

HERBS FOR TOPICAL USE

Skin is your biggest organ and you can benefit as much from the healing benefits of herbs by applying them to your skin, as you would if you took them as a tincture or a capsule. Actually, it's safer to use herbs topically because that way they do not interfere with other medication you may be taking. Medicinal herbs can be applied to different areas of the body, eg nose, genitals, anus, mouth and gums, wounds, eyes, sprains, skin-rash, etc.

Herbs for topical use can be prepared in many different ways. Sometimes, all you need to do is use the fresh leaves or flowers and rub them on your skin. However, this may work against mosquitos (basil leaves) or insect stings (comfrey leaves) but in case of a specific health problem, herbs need to be prepared in a way that turns them into a herbal remedy, eg as a cream, lotion, poultice, etc.

16 types of topical applications:

1. Infusion

A strong herbal brew (as explained above).

2. Tincture

Dried or fresh herbs are steeped in alcohol or water. The alcohol not only extracts the plant's active ingredients, it also serves as a preservative. A tincture will keep for two years. Tinctures should be made from individual herbs. If you need to mix them, you can do so with the already prepared tinctures.

3. Infused oil

Herbs' active ingredients can be extracted in oil and used in massage oils, creams, and ointments. Oil can be infused in two ways: the hot method (suitable for comfrey, chickweed, and rosemary) and the cold method (suitable for calendula and St. John's Wort).

4. Cream

A cream is a mixture of water and oils. It softens the skin and is easily absorbed by the skin. Home-made creams will last for only several months but their shelf life can be extended by keeping them in a fridge or by adding a few drops of a preservative.

5. Compress

A compress promotes the healing of wounds and muscle injuries. It is used by soaking a cloth in hot herbal extract and applying it to the painful area. However, for a headache, you should use a cold compress. You can also use infusions, decoctions, and tinctures for a compress by diluting them with water.

6. Poultice

This is similar to a compress except that instead of using only the liquid, the whole herb is used. Poultices are usually applied hot. You soak whole leaves in hot water. After a while, you drain them and apply them to painful areas.

7. Decoction

This method is used to extract a plant's active ingredients from roots, barks, twigs, and some berries. The herb is put in cold water and simmered on low heat for one hour.

8. Vaginal douche

Douching is washing or flushing the vagina with water or other fluids. Vaginal douches usually contain vinegar, baking soda, or iodine. You can get them from pharmacies; however, most doctors do not agree with this practice as it upsets the natural balance of bacteria in the vagina.

9. Sitz bath

A sitz bath is a warm, shallow bath used to provide relief from pain, itching, and irritation in the genital area. . Different soothing or antimicrobial herbs can be added to a sitz bath. For example, you can try using 1 cup of each - witch hazel bark or leaves, yarrow, calendula, uva ursi, plantain, lavender, etc. Put them in a big bowl, pour over 2 liters of hot water, and let it steep for 20 minutes. Fill the tub with enough water so that your genitals are covered and add the infusion of herbs. If you don't have all of the herbs, you can use only some of them. There are many other herbs you can use and this partly depends on the symptoms you are experiencing.

10.   Linament

Linament is a skin rub. It is usually used to relieve pain and stiffness, eg muscular pain, strains, arthritis, etc.

11.   Lotion

The lotion is a topical remedy with low viscosity, ie it has low water content. It is applied to the skin with bare hands, a brush, a clean cloth, or cotton wool. Lotions are usually cosmetic products, rather than medical ones (eg hand lotion, suntan lotion, etc).

12.   Ointment

An ointment is similar to cream but contains no water. It consists only of oils or fats. It does not blend with the skin but forms a protective layer over it. Good for protecting the skin from moisture (eg nappy rash).

13.   Essential oils

Essential oil is basically the essence of a flower. These oils have many therapeutic applications and are usually used diluted with carrier oils.

Herbalism developed locally which explains why herbs used in Chinese Traditional Medicine, Africa, or Europe often differ. Not all plants grow everywhere so healers had to make do with what was available locally.

This is why it's impossible to make a list of the best herbs for topical use as those used in Western herbal medicine differ from those used in South America or Africa. However, as TCM, Ayurveda, and South American herbs may not be available everywhere, we decided to list herbs commonly used for topical applications that are easily available and that are not difficult to grow or wildcraft throughout North America, Europe, and Central Asia.

<u>13 best herbs for topical use:</u>
1. Arnica
2. Lavender
3. St. John's wort
4. Chamomile
5. Yarrow
6. Calendula
7. Plaintain

8. Comfrey
9. Capsicum
10. Eucalyptus
11. Thyme
12. Oregano

An important aspect of holistic health is prevention. Not only do we live in a very polluted world, we also willingly absorb a lot of toxins from the cosmetic and household cleaning products we use every day (this is particularly true of women).

These products often contain harmful ingredients and this only adds up to the toxic load most of us already carry. Find out about nontoxic and organic products you could use instead of what you've been using until now. Besides, there are easy ways to make at least some of these products at home, eg toothpaste, facial creams and masks, lip gloss, shampoo, cleaning products, etc.

SMOKABLE HERBS

Herbs are usually used orally or topically. But we often forget that another way of benefitting from their healing properties is by smoking or steam inhalation. Herbs are smoked to relax, destress, or provide a hallucinogenic experience. Some have antipsychotic properties while others can induce an alternate state of mind. Strangely enough, smoking herbs can also help you lose weight or quit smoking. Besides, herbs with sedative or pain-killing properties were often given to women during labor (Fenugreek, Black Cohosh, Raspberry Leaf, etc).

Most people think of cannabis when they think about smokable herbs but dozens of other herbs can be smoked. Not all of them will get you high or induce hallucinations, nor will they make you an addict. This means they are perfectly safe and legal to use both at home and in public. It's best to use these mild herbs in a blend with other, stronger herbs. However, regardless of their strength, they all provide relaxation.

HERBS COMMONLY USED FOR SMOKING BLENDS

- *Blue lotus*

Blue lots will easily relax you. It is used for its aphrodisiac and sedative effects. It is very calming.

- *Damiana*

Damiana is also commonly smoked for its aphrodisiac qualities and is often added to blends.

- *White sage*

When smoked, white sage can boost your mood and memory and is very relaxing. It can also help clear your lungs, throat, and sinuses.

- *Dagga*

The wild dagga is very similar to cannabis. It has a sedative and calming effect. It can boost your mood and mental clarity and will have an amazing effect on your color perception.

- *Passionflower*

Passionflower is often mixed with damiana. It is a very relaxing herb and is often smoked to help relieve anxiety and insomnia.

- *Mullein*

Mullein is a common base for smoking blends as it's neutral and very light. Smoking mullein can help you clear your lungs.

- *Catnip*

When smoked, it has a slightly hypnotic effect so can help with insomnia. Fantastic herb for relaxation.

- *Red Raspberry*

Red Raspberry leaves are usually mixed with Uva Ursi and Damiana. This combination adds great flavor to your smoking mix. Besides, smoking red raspberry can help stabilize your blood sugar levels

- *Coltsfoot*

The main benefit of smoking this herb is that it helps you get rid of phlegm.

- *Mugwort*

Mugwort was often used in religious or spiritual ceremonies. It is known to promote vivid dreams. The smoke also has a mild psychotropic effect, as does the steam when this herb is being boiled.

- *Uva Ursi*

Uva Ursi herb was very popular with Native Americans and was regularly used for ceremonial purposes.

- *Skullcap*

Skullcap is mild and very calming.

There are many herbal blends to choose from but if you are serious about smoking herbs, you should learn how to make your own blend. It's not difficult and can be a lot of fun if you have access to fresh herbs.

TIPS ON HOW TO MAKE YOUR OWN SMOKING BLEND:

- Harvest fresh, young herbs
- Dry the leaves slowly indoors (you can hang them out or spread them in a thin layer)
- When completely dry, crush the leaves by hand
- Combine several herbs to make your own blend (eg mullein is a good base and should represent about 50% of the blend). Add other herbs for the "body" of the blend (about 40%) and add some flavoring herbs, eg sage (about 10%).
- Store your blend in a glass jar or a resealable plastic pouch

CHAPTER 7
HERB COMBINATIONS

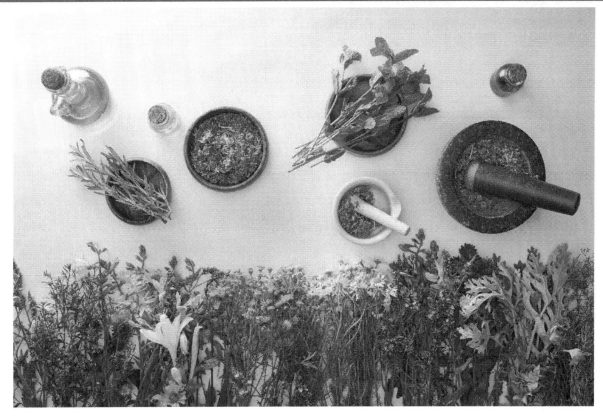

Herbs have been used to support our health since time immemorial. We often support our various organs unknowingly by following a diet rich in nutrient-dense foods (eg oregano). However, people usually start taking herbs seriously only once they become aware of their numerous health benefits. Unfortunately, this usually happens only once their health has been compromised. Another reason for the growing interest in herbal remedies is that many strains of bacteria have become resistant to antibiotics. That's why people are now turning to nature in search of time-tested, non-toxic medication.

In this chapter, we will look at herbs that support the pancreas, kidneys, liver, respiratory organs, and colon. What will immediately become obvious is that certain herbs have so many active ingredients, they benefit almost all the organs, eg dandelion, licorice, horsetail, etc.

HERBS FOR PANCREAS AND KIDNEY SUPPORT

The pancreas is an organ that produces enzymes and hormones that aid digestion. Its proper functioning is particularly important for diabetics. Fortunately, there are many herbs that not only protect the pancreas from disease but help restore it in case it has become inflamed, ie in the case of pancreatitis.

Herbs helpful in maintaining and restoring pancreatic health include:

- **Licorice root**

Anti-inflammatory properties of licorice can help reduce the pain and swelling that is typical of pancreatitis.

- **Goldenseal**

This herb supports the pancreas by lowering blood sugar levels which is particularly beneficial to diabetics.

- **Horsetail**

One of the consequences of pancreatitis is that its tissue gets broken. Horsetail helps regenerate it.

- **Oregano**

Oregano is an excellent natural remedy for hyperglycemia as well as many other complications that result from diabetes.

- **Dandelion**

Dandelion root extract (tincture) kills pancreatic cancer cells even when nothing else seems to work. Besides, dandelion root tea is an efficient natural remedy for flushing toxins out of the body which helps restore the damaged pancreatic tissues.

- **Gentian**

Gentian roots remedies improve digestion by boosting the production of pancreatic enzymes.

- **Olive leaves**

Consistent use of olive leaf extract (tincture) will improve the overall functioning of the pancreas. It will also reduce the pain and swelling caused by pancreatitis and protects the pancreas from the damage caused by free radicals. Consistent use will significantly lower your risk of pancreatic cancer.

Another organ essential to your overall health are the kidneys. Their main function is to filter the blood and they do this by removing waste from the body (mainly urea). They also regulate the body's water volume and salt content. Chronic kidney disease, ie the gradual loss of kidney function, is a life-threatening condition. Sadly, many people are unaware their kidneys are rapidly degenerating. The main causes of this condition are diabetes and high blood pressure.

The best herbs to support your kidneys include:

- **Horsetail**

Valued for its diuretic properties that help flush out the urinary tract and kidneys.

- **Green tea**

Recommended to everyone whose kidneys are not functioning properly because of its powerful anti-inflammatory and diuretic properties. It also contains polyphenols that prevent the formation of kidney stones.

- **Hydrangea root**

A great herb to support your bladder and kidney health. Prevents the kidney stones from forming by helping the body use calcium so there is no surplus the body turns to kidney stones.

- **Couch grass**

This herb will increase your urine production which will indirectly help you solve some of your urinary tract infections – the more often you urinate, the more likely you are to flush out the pathogens. Couch grass can also help dissolve kidney stones.

- **Goldenrod**

This is a well-known folk remedy for urinary tract problems, including malfunctioning kidneys.

- **Chanca Piedra**

The name means "stone breaker". This is the most popular herb throughout South America when it comes to getting rid of kidney stones naturally.

- **Java tea**

Drinking Java tea will not only help you keep your kidneys healthy, it will also help you dissolve kidney stones and cure kidney infections.

- **Dandelion**

Dandelion is a strong diuretic and a very efficient natural remedy for kidney detox. Consistent use will help dissolve kidney stones.

- **Celery root**

Both the root and the seeds have diuretic properties and are recommended to everyone with urinary tract problems.

HERBS FOR LIVER SUPPORT

The liver is one of your key organs because it helps you stay free of toxins. It constantly processes the waste that gets into our system from the environment, diet, or unhealthy living habits. A liver that's no longer functioning properly may be the cause of many other health conditions, eg frequent headaches, chronic fatigue, hormonal problems, nervous system disorders, kidney problems, cirrhosis, jaundice, hepatitis, etc.

So, to stay healthy, you need to take very good care of your liver and support it in any way we can. If you can't reduce the toxic load, at least include the herbs that support liver health in your diet.

Liver-supporting herbs include:

- **Dandelion**

Dandelion leaves extract (tincture) supports the liver due to its powerful antioxidant and anti-inflammatory properties. Herbal remedies made from dandelion root and leaves have been successfully used to fight cirrhosis and fatty liver for hundreds of years.

- **Chicory root**

Chickory root is a well- known folk remedy for liver disorders. Even ancient Egyptians used it to cleanse both the blood and the liver. It helps with the production of bile which makes fat be broken down more quickly.

- **Milk thistle**

Milk thistle is possibly the best-known natural remedy for liver conditions. It promotes detox, increases bile production, and regenerates the liver.

- **Licorice**

Licorice contains compounds that help fight hepatitis and cancer. The licorice root is particularly efficient for liver detox.

- **Yellow dock root**

Yellow dock root tonic is an excellent remedy for many liver problems. It encourages detox and stimulates the production of bile which improves both digestion and overall liver health.

HERBS FOR RESPIRATORY SUPPORT

Respiratory conditions affect the lungs and respiratory system (both upper and lower). These are usually not serious conditions but if they become chronic, they can lead to pneumonia and long-term damage to the respiratory tract.

Antibiotics have been the common therapy for respiratory problems. However, although they provided quick relief from the symptoms, the long-term use of antibiotics contributed to the development of antibiotic-resistant strains. On the other hand, herbal remedies take longer to act but are as effective and come with no side effects.

Common herbal remedies for respiratory problems include:

- **Licorice**

Licorice has significant antibacterial, antiviral, expectorant, anti-inflammatory properties which is why it is an excellent folk remedy for reducing inflammation of the respiratory organs.

- **Echinacea**

Being high in antioxidants, echinacea is an efficient natural remedy for many conditions of the respiratory system (eg bronchitis).

- **Ginko**

Ginkgo is one of the best herbal remedies for preventing asthma attacks. It can quickly soothe coughing and wheezing and help you breathe normally and easily.

- **Mullein**

Mullein is not often recommended for respiratory infections but its extract has powerful anti-inflammatory and antioxidant properties that eliminate mucus. Mullein tea can soothe the inflammation of respiratory organs but you shouldn't take more than one cup a day.

- **Thyme**

Thyme has antibiotic, antiviral, and anti-fungal properties so there is almost no respiratory condition it cannot help with. You can take it as tea or tincture but it's particularly potent when used as an essential oil.

- **Oregano**

Oregano is also an effective remedy for respiratory infections. It will kill bacteria and clear mucus. You can take it as tea or you can use a diluted essential oil.

- **Cannabis**

Cannabis has anti-inflammatory properties which you can benefit from if you are struggling with respiratory conditions. The reason vaporized cannabis makes breathing easier is because it makes your respiratory tract expand.

- **Chaparral**

Chaparral tincture has significant antibacterial, decongestant, and antihistamine properties that can help with many respiratory infections.

HERBS FOR COLON CLEANSE

Colon cleansing is another word for flushing the waste from a colon. This has been a common practice for thousands of years.

However, although a colon cleanse comes with many benefits, it also brings certain risks. An alternative to colon flushing in a hospital is using herbs in the form of teas, capsules, or powders. Many herbs are natural laxatives and act anti-inflammatory.

The common herbs that can cleanse your colon naturally include:

- **Cascara Sagrada**

Cascara Sagrada is a gentle laxative and is often used for natural colon cleansing.

- **Senna**

Powerful laxative, Senna tea or capsules should not be used for more than a few consecutive days.

- **Phyllium**

The seeds and husk of psyllium are a well-known folk remedy for colon cleansing. What makes it such an efficient laxative is a certain type of fiber it contains, called mucilage, which absorbs water in the digestive tract.

- **Fennel**

Fennel seeds and root aid digestion and prevent colics. Often combined with laxatives, eg rhubarb or senna. On its own, it's mild enough to give to children.

- **Barberry bark**

This herb supports colon health by promoting bile flow and acting as a natural laxative.

OTHER BOOKS IN SAME SERIES

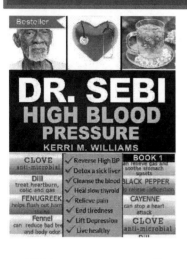 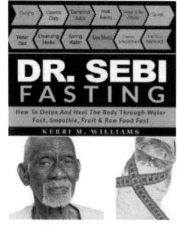 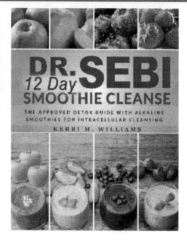

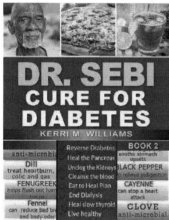 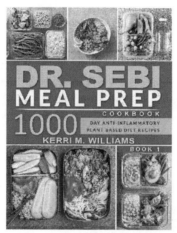 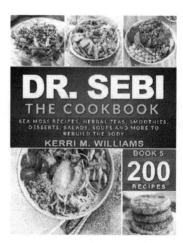

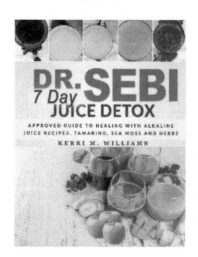 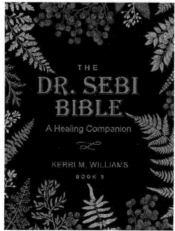 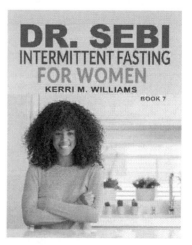

Made in the USA
Monee, IL
05 October 2021